Spiritual Healing

Reiki Guide to Increase Energy, Improve Health, and Feel Amazing With Reiki Healing

(Ancient Healing Power to Increase Energy, Awaken Chakras and Improve Health)

Paula Stiene

Published by Rob Miles

Paula Stiene

All Rights Reserved

Spiritual Healing: Reiki Guide to Increase Energy, Improve Health, and Feel Amazing With Reiki Healing (Ancient Healing Power to Increase Energy, Awaken Chakras and Improve Health)

ISBN 978-1-989990-26-1

All rights reserved. No part of this guide may be reproduced in any form without permission in writing from the publisher except in the case of brief quotations embodied in critical articles or reviews.

Legal & Disclaimer

The information contained in this book is not designed to replace or take the place of any form of medicine or professional medical advice. The information in this book has been provided for educational and entertainment purposes only.

The information contained in this book has been compiled from sources deemed reliable, and it is accurate to the best of the Author's knowledge; however, the Author cannot guarantee its accuracy and validity and cannot be held liable for any errors or omissions. Changes are periodically made to this book. You must consult your doctor or get professional medical advice before using any of the suggested remedies, techniques, or information in this book.

Upon using the information contained in this book, you agree to hold harmless the Author from and against any damages, costs, and expenses, including any legal fees potentially resulting from the application of any of the information provided by this guide. This disclaimer applies to any damages or injury caused by the use and application, whether directly or indirectly, of any advice or information presented, whether for breach of contract, tort, negligence, personal injury, criminal intent, or under any other cause of action.

You agree to accept all risks of using the information presented inside this book. You need to consult a professional medical practitioner in order to ensure you are both able and healthy enough to participate in this program.

Table of Contents

INTRODUCTION 1

CHAPTER 1: UNIVERSAL ENERGY IN HUMAN BODY 3

CHAPTER 2: REIKI HANDS POSITIONS FOR SELF TREATMENT 9

CHAPTER 3: RELAXING WITH REIKI. 19

CHAPTER 4: THE VARIOUS SORTS OF REIKI 27

CHAPTER 5: BENEFITS OF REIKI MEDITATION 47

CHAPTER 6: ARE THERE SAFETY CONCERNS ABOUT THE USE OF REIKI? 56

CHAPTER 7: ANIMAL HEALER SECTION 68

CHAPTER 8: MEDITATION IN PREPARATION FOR HEALING 75

CHAPTER 9: INDIVIDUAL ELEMENTS 89

CHAPTER 10: EXCITING TIMES 102

CHAPTER 11: REIKI & STRESS RELIEF 118

CHAPTER 12: MENTAL AND EMOTIONAL HEALING 131

CHAPTER 13: SYMBOLS OF REIKI 147

CHAPTER 14: IMPROVING YOUR ABILITY TO CHANNEL REIKI ENERGY 157

CHAPTER 15: SELF HEALING- HEALING YOURSELF, BEFORE HEALING OTHERS 171

CHAPTER 16: FROM PATIENT TO PRACTITIONER 188

CONCLUSION 192

Introduction

Reiki is a very old method of healing that has been in use and still is being used by several people and practitioners around the globe where palms of the hands are used to do the healing. It was founded in India many years ago, even before the birth of Jesus Christ or Buddha. The names that were used to term Reiki were lost during as time went by because of the methods of relaying knowledge, passing down the knowledge from one generation to another by the use of word of mouth only.

This healing art, later on, got lost completely because of the poor transition of passage to the different generations but luckily it was rediscovered by a Japanese monk called Dr.Mikao Usui, and he was the one that named the healing art, REIKI. Reiki is a Japanese word which when cut into two, it means universal life energy,

RYE means universal, and KEY means life energy.

Reiki is everywhere, being present in all places at the same time. It is the consciousness that is spiritual, deep within consciousness that is given by the higher power. On the other hand, Ki is a unique energy, the unexplainable energy because it is of a higher power that can give life to all living organisms.

The KI energy can be channeled to a healing power that can be able to heal by the use of certain techniques and also be able to preserve life. Ki energy has different positive impacts on our bodies. For instance, when you feel your body is functioning well, your body is not in pain, hurt or any sort of tiredness, this means that the KI energy is flowing well that is why you are feeling enthusiastic and healthy.

This book is for anyone interested in the art of Reiki healing.

Chapter 1: Universal Energy In Human Body

The force of life is a subtle energy that flows and surrounds routes, such as chakras and meridians, and it is ever present in all living beings. The vital force nourishes and encourages the functioning of all cells of the body. If your life force is low, you will probably feel brittle. You're likely to be sick. Enhancing your strength in life will help your body heal and remain healthy. Your life force flow becomes disrupted, causing your body organs to function diminished. If you have adverse ideas or adverse emotions about yourself, your general body balance (mental, emotional and physical) will be troubled, then you get sick. Thoughts and emotions have an immense impact on life force.

It is the inspiration for our whole existence. In truth, the warm temperature of the sun that heats our bodies, the gasoline that we use in our car, the power used inside the household, is the same energy forms. It is the energy that sustains life, providing vital energy to all living systems. The whole Universe, starting from the stars in the sky to the atoms that create them, including the world we live in and our bodies, everything we see or do, is made up of the Universal Energy, at the most fundamental level.

Sensitive To The Atmospheric Energy

Our souls can feel the universal vibrations been more aware of the energy present around. They tend to sense the power of the surroundings and even that of people who aren't associated with them. Because the planet's vibration keeps increasing, more individuals are becoming receptive to the regular strength that surrounds us. Right here are seven indications that you are an amazing delicate empath for the Universal Energy:

1. Sensitive To Other Humans' Feelings

Empaths can often assume what another individual feels, and they can even perceive their feelings as though they were theirs. They can also tell you what someone else feels, even if that person isn't there with them.

This can be arduous, which is why protecting their power is very essential to an empath. There are plenty of signs of survival for empaths and extremely sensitive people to help prevent and alleviate an emotional overload.

2. Feeling Uncomfortable In Enclosed Spaces Or Crowded Areas

Empaths might also be overwhelmed and probably barely agitated while in a crowded space or even in some public locations. This is because the human beings around them are connected to them and there is an inflow of energy.

Empaths and highly sensitive people (HSP) are also more aware of their environment, which means that certain sounds, smells, and lights can be overwhelming for them.

This can be difficult to solve, which is why it is important for empaths and highly sensitive people to develop protective tools.

3. A Very Good Intuition

Since empathy is so aware of the setting and other people's energy, their instinct is often very powerful. Before an event happens, they can comprehend it and can experience when someone they care about is going through a difficult moment.

4. Looking For Spiritual Connection

People who are more sensitive to the Universal Energy have a profound desire to find a spiritual link with their partner, establish their spiritual family, or even a home with which they can resonate profoundly on a deep psychological level.

5. Strong Desires

Empaths have very vibrant and excessive objectives, complete of creativity that they often maintain in mind. A chance to visit other places is a dream come true for such individuals to explore other levels of reality.

6. Experience Growth In Their Inner Self

Empaths are prepared to open their minds at any time to see the world from many angles because of their empathy, creativity, and a willingness to learn more about their soul's requirements.

Via different reports along with gaining access to kundalini electricity or opening the third eye, they regularly experience spiritual awakenings.

7. Non-Stop Search Of The Reason For Existence

For empaths, life is not just about work, family, material security, or simply seeking pleasure. They feel that life is something much bigger and deeper and they spend a lot of time reflecting on its true meaning.

Empaths attempt to incorporate themselves and create their private contributions in a consistent and beneficial manner into the planet. Since this strategy can become their life's symbolic value, they may sometimes feel disgusted by someone who does not share this perspective.

To Develop & Nurture Your Sensitivity to the Universal Energy

Examine and evaluate the various seasons of the year and the lunar stages of your mental states.

Have a paper and write down your most vivid dreams and make sure you're perusing it regularly.

Attempt to discover patterns that are showing up regularly. This will assist you to interpret and discover a deeper significance in your dreams.

Mediate more to feel the power of all living humans, particularly in nature, and how things are interconnected.

Observing the sky and star-looking practice deepens your link to the world.

Chapter 2: Reiki Hands Positions For Self Treatment

Reiki conveys an all-encompassing way to deal with recuperating and regards the body in general. A Reiki treatment is utilized to adjust the energies, which assists with recuperating at diverse levels, for example, physical, mental and otherworldly.

Amid a Reiki session different sensations may be felt, for example, warmth, icy or shivering in the hands. On the other hand, it might be that you won't encounter any of these. This is not a reason for concern as every session is diverse. Reiki will dependably work, paying little respect to what you may, or may not, be feeling.

Utilizing the different hand positions accurately is critical as they cover the greater part of the principle areas of the body. They can likewise be utilized to regard yourself and additionally others. Clearly, there are slight contrasts close by positions on the off chance that you are treating yourself, as opposed to treating another person. Continuously be aware of individual protection and unseemly touching when treating another individual. Reiki vitality will work pretty much also without utilizing direct contact.

The hand positions beneath spread the nuts and bolts for treating another individual. To utilize them for self-treatment you will need to adjust them in like manner. For example, in position one, your palms would be drop down the face and guiding towards your crown.

Position 1:

Place your hands fit as a fiddle, parallel to one side and right of the nose. Your palms ought to be at the highest point of the forehead confronting towards the feet.

Position 2:

Your hands ought to be set on the sanctuaries with the fingertips coming to the cheekbones.

Position 3:

One hand ought to be set over every ear fit as a fiddle with the fingers confronting towards the feet.

Position 4:

Tenderly grasp the back of the head keeping them together and confronting towards the feet.

Position 5:

Place your hands covering the front of the neck with the fingers directing towards the feet. Make a point not to touch the neck as this can be uncomfortable for a few individuals.

Position 6:

Remaining to the right side, put your hands in a T-shape at the highest point of the breastbone, simply under the neck.

Your left hand forms the highest point of the T with your right hand directing towards the feet.

Position 7:

Keeping focused right side, move your hands to the center of the midsection area. Your hands ought to be set indicating over the body with the abandoned hand the privilege.

Position 8:

Next move your hands to simply beneath the navel, keeping the deserted hand the privilege.

Position 9:

For this position your fingers need to point towards the feet. Your hands ought to form a V over the pelvic bone.

Position 10:

Presently move down to the knee area. Glass your hands around every knee thus.

Position 11:

Rehash with respect to the knees yet over the lower legs.

Position 12:

The last position is for the feet. Just place your hands tenderly over the soles of the feet and hold.

Positions 5 - 9 can likewise be utilized on the back of the other individual to completely finish the treatment.

On the off chance that conceivable, attempt to hold every position for more or less three minutes before moving to the following one as this permits the vitality to stream bringing more positive results from the treatment.

Reiki Hands Position for Treating Other

There are 12 customary Usui Reiki hand positions for the front of the body. Reiki Practitioners utilize these positions as a beginning stage for a natural session. Ordinarily they don't utilize the positions in a definite request in light of the fact that naturally their hands are guided to focuses on the body where Reiki is generally required. In Reiki sessions, hand positions typically start at the head. They build up a feeling of offset through the entire body. These hand positions treat the mind which influences whatever is left of the body.

HAND POSITION #1 EYES AND FACE - hands are set over shut eyes with hands to every side of the nose and fingertips laying on the cheekbones, thumbs lay on the third eye chakra. A tissue can be put over the face for comfort, or hands can drift two or three inches over the face. A few individuals lean toward this technique in light of the fact that the Reiki expert's hands are warm. This position makes an extremely unwinding state which is similar to being in the middle of waking and dozing.

HAND POSITION #2 TOP OF HEAD - spot hands silly (close to the back) of the head with fingers indicating down the ears and wrists touching. On the off chance that the beneficiary has a unique haircut, drift your hands in this position simply over the head.

HAND POSITION #3 TEMPLES - spot hands on sanctuaries with writs laying on both side of forehead between the eyebrows and hairlines, finger touching the cheekbones. This position helps in adjusting the cerebrum and diminishes migraines. Helps individuals join profoundly.

HAND POSITION #4 EARS - spot hands over ears. This position treats ears, listening to and jaws. Supports harmony and calms occupied personalities.

HAND POSITON #5 BACK OF HEAD - spot hands under head, fingers indicating the neck. Move head to the other side, put one hand under; move head to other side, place other hand under. Hold base of head with fingers simply touching the highest point of neck. This position treats the third eye 6th chakra and the back of the head.

HAND POSITION #6 THROAT - hold face and container the button with fingers close however not touching the throat. This position treats the throat fifth chakra. Helps correspondence issues and treats hypertension.

HAND POSITION #7 COLLARBONE - spot hands on the sides of the neck with fingers over collarbone indicating the focal point of midsection. Treats the thymus organ which is critical for safe capacity.

HAND POSITION #8 BACK OF NECK AND FRONT OF HEART - place one hand underneath neck and the other hand over the heart fingers indicating down. Treats the throat fifth chakra and the heart fourth chakra at the same time. Helps expression and talking reality. Is likewise useful for hypertension.

HAND POSITION #9 HEART - spot delivers a "T", one hand on a level plane over the bosoms and one hand vertically between the bosoms. Treats the heart fourth chakra and all things connected with the heart, circulatory framework, veins and corridors, and lungs. At the point when the heart chakra is opened, the supporting impacts of love are more claimed and additionally the capacity to experience forgiveness and sympathy.

HAND POSITION #10 UPPER ABDOMEN - spot turns in a line on the upper stomach area. Treats the sun oriented plexus third chakra which helps the digestive organs, stomach, gallbladder, entrails, liver, and spleen. Assists with diabetes, liver sickness and gastrointestinal issues.

HAND POSITION #11 MIDDLE ABDOMEN - spot hands on a level plane, one hand above navel and one hand beneath navel. Treats pancreas, gallbladder and guts.

HAND POSITION #12 LOWER ABDOMEN - spot hands on lower midriff. Avoid genital area. Treats sacral second chakra which helps regenerative organs, bladder and pelvic area. Additionally empowers the "hara", Japanese word importance focus of the body's vitality. Helps imagination, sexuality, and feelings.

Chapter 3: Relaxing With Reiki.

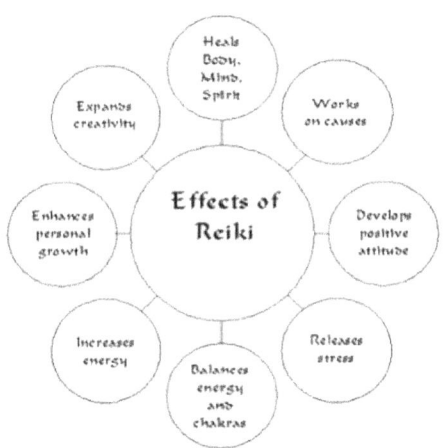

Are you still skeptical that Reiki can actually help you relax? That's absolutely fine! You may already do relaxation techniques that let you think more clearly, work through knotty problems or just clear your mind and ease cramped muscles before you start or end your day. Reiki is just one more kind of relaxation technique you can employ to do all of those and much more.

You may be familiar with Yoga, deep breathing, biofeedback, meditation, Tai

Chi or the devotions and prayers of your religious beliefs. Even walking, running, and gardening can be techniques that help you to relax and re-center yourself when you are feeling mentally tangled up.

As we discussed earlier, Reiki is simply manipulating the life force energy that flows through your body and this helps you relax. Just like the river flowing smoothly when there are no huge boulders near the surface, your life force energy will flow smoothly through your cells and organs. It will help you think more rationally and easily and you'll be able to make decisions more readily. Or perhaps you are anxious about a test you have to take or a speech you have been asked to make. Reiki will help with any anxiety you might feel in those situations.

Reiki helps even when you don't expect it

Should everything be going quite well in your life, you might wonder how Reiki will be of help to you. When I heard about Reiki, I was in perfect health both physically and mentally so I wondered just how Reiki could help me. Actually, I found out that I was under stress and didn't even know it! All those little things you might not even think about put stress upon your body and mind causing little ripples in the energies that flows through you. It's just like one boulder near the surface of that smoothly flowing river disturbs the easy movement of the water.

When it comes to doubts

When you have your first Reiki session, if you have some doubts about the treatment, it may not work as well as you think it should. This could be a result of your skepticism since mind over matter really is a bigger deal than most people think. It is important to believe that Reiki works in order to get the most out of the treatment. If you doubt, you are shorting yourself out of some great benefits, though you will certainly still getting some good energy flow. Even if you do not think you are getting results, you can be assured that it has had *some* result that will help you detect the effect of the process in your second Reiki treatment.

During your first session you may feel nothing physically but many have reported feeling warmth throughout their bodies no matter where the practitioner's hands are placed. Others have said they felt vibrations or just deep relaxation. The more accepting you are about the procedure, the more you will feel and be able to follow as your therapist performs the treatment. No matter what you feel, when the session is over, you will have a sense of well-being and refreshment with a more positive outlook on the world.

What to expect at the first session

Reiki practitioners want you to be comfortable so the process can be performed anywhere, though the quieter the surroundings, the better. Whomever you choose to receive a treatment from will be very attentive to your comfort and will not usually request any paperwork to be filled out like your personal physician may. The most you may have to do is sign a waiver giving them permission to perform the procedure. Most likely you will be asked if you have any health conditions that would interfere with your ability to lay flat on your back since Reiki works best when your body can completely relax.

The therapy room will probably look similar to a massage therapy room in many aspects, though the examination or treatment table won't necessarily have the hole for your face as a massage table does. If you aren't able to lay on your back then you may be asked to sit in a comfortable, supportive chair. You will not be asked to undress for your first session and subsequent treatments may or may not require partial or full disrobing, depending upon what you are receiving treatment for.

Music is often played to mask ambient sounds that might disturb you during your session. If you have a specific type of music that helps you relax or that you prefer when you meditate, you can usually request your Reiki therapist to play it during your procedure. Below is an example of how your therapy room may look. There is usually a single table rather than two unless you and a companion are receiving treatments together.

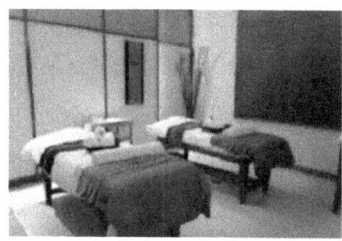

A normal Reiki session often consists of a light touch or hovering of the practitioner's hands on or over the head, face, front and back of your torso. The 6 chakra regions will be the primary focus, but the practitioner may focus on other areas as well if he feels led to do so. There is not usually any pressure brought to bear on those portions the therapist touches, similar to just resting your hand on those parts of your body. Your therapist will be conscientious about being sure that you do not experience physical or mental discomfort. The placement of the therapist's hands should never feel intrusive or inappropriate since this will cause adverse electrical impulses that will block the positive energy the Reiki attempts to impart.

As mentioned before, Reiki is simply a practitioner laying hands on portions of your body to help the energies contained within you to flow smoothly. However, some massage therapists are also trained and certified to practice Reiki and may incorporate both sets of training in any session after your first.

It may seem silly to go to someone just to get help relaxing, but without these types of techniques then you may not be fully relaxed. If you don't know how to do it on your own, then you need someone else to help you with it. When you find the person you want to give you Reiki, be sure to let them know everything that will make you comfortable. This is *your* special time and your therapist is there to make you feel wonderful. If you need a pillow beneath your knees or a blanket, if laying on your back or stomach is uncomfortable or if you don't care to be touched in specific places due to tender scar tissue from surgery or other physical injury – be sure to tell your therapist. It is their job to make you comfortable. If you are comfortable, the easier their job will be.

Chapter 4: The Various Sorts Of Reiki

Crystals are made use of either around the client or on different Chakra factors, or held by either the Therapist or the recipient throughout a recovery session.

Saku Reiki - is thought about a detailed kind of Reiki where the expert utilizes a detailed system of recovery approaches. This kind of Reiki is made use of lots of times when western medication isn't really as efficient for an individual.

This system of Reiki is assumed that recovery comes from within. Dragon Reiki promotes recovery of the spirit and also the physical body since it is thought that just when the spirit is in equilibrium as well as consistency that physical recovery could take place.

Shamanic Reiki- This kind of Reiki includes both Reiki and also Shamanic techniques. Generally in different societies, a witch doctor is one that is mentally skilled in their society's devoutness. Human beings grow on meaning, habits as well as patterns as well as Reiki has these aspects.

An additional attribute special to Egyptian Reiki is the adverse power drainpipe. Due to the fact that this kind of Reiki is reliable for that it is a spiritual recovery Reiki.

Several times the transfer of power could be really felt from the expert to the recipient. Numerous conventional western physicians are currently including Reiki right into their clinical techniques to improve the recovery and also state of being in their people.

This is a quite effective sign as well as could be utilized either methods for recovery functions. Both means work in cleaning up the Chakras.

One means the Fire Snake could be made use of to ground the individual as well as to remove the individual of unfavorable power with the physical bodies last Chakra as it is removed via the Chakra course. It is the Reiki master that identifies just how the Fire Snake will certainly be utilized to ideal deal with the recipient throughout a session. This sign is utilized to make sure that the recipient is hip to appropriately to the recovery power.

The recovery power of Reiki and also the crystals are made use of with each other to impact a recovery procedure in the recipient. In enhancement to the routine concerns like all Reiki addresses crystal recovery with Reiki is likewise valuable for kinds of psychosomatic health problems such as migraine headaches, frustrations, acid indigestion, cranky bowel disorder and also bronchial asthma.

As an outcome, there are various kinds of Reiki. The different kinds of Reiki offered today integrate the conventional kind of Reiki recovery with various other aspects as improvements. Maintain in mind no matter of the kind of Reiki one techniques it entails funneling global power and also after that giving it in an individual in demand of recovery liking one's self.

The individual obtaining an Angelic Reiki Therapy has actually modification brought to them by eliminating old idea kinds that are not in conformity with Magnificent resonances. As an organic recovery device, it additionally assists to recover those points that are inscribed on us from the previously.

Fire Snake Reiki- The therapists in this system make use of the signs of the Fire Snake to recover the recipient both literally and also emotionally. One of the major factors that the Fire Snake is made use of is to open up the recipient's chakras. The master therapist might be offered the expertise that the individual is not prepared for this kind of therapy as well as will certainly make use of one more kind of recovery sign to open up one or 2 chakras just for a recovery session.

Dragon Reiki- This is amongst one of the most preferred kind of Reiki today. It integrates the recovery homes of the Dragon in Chinese Devoutness along with their Typical Medicines. In Chinese Devoutness the dragon has solid recovery residential properties and also connect to nature.

Old Egyptian Reiki- standard Reiki acquires its power from a global greater power resource; Ancient Egyptian Reiki regulates this power and also transforms it right into solid recovery resonances. The distinction in between standard Reiki and also Egyptian Reiki is it uses power from the planet.

Usui Reiki- This is thought about the typical kind or Reiki that Dr. Usui presented to the remainder of the globe. If an individual is offered Usui Reiki it recovers them on numerous degrees; literally, mentally, psychologically and also mentally. Over the years the recovery fine art of Reiki has actually been instructed and also spread out vocally.

If one runs out equilibrium mentally one could not anticipate to recover literally. As the recipient starts to recover emotionally outward initial after that the physical body does just what the divinities forecast it to do and also recovery beginnings. The therapist of this method has the capacity to absorb love and also power from the greater resource and also stations it to the recipient to recover them mentally.

Among the differences in between typical Reiki and also Dragon Reiki is that some sign or photo of a Dragon exists which aids the therapist in routing the Dragon power to the client. Before a Dragon Reiki session, the recipient should remove their minds as well as spirits so their spirits could obtain the powers that the Dragon and also the Greater Powers need to over them.

Like conventional recovery Angelic Reiki likewise has the choice of range recovery and also self-healing. Rather of signs, the professional utilizes the angelic power to attune the recipient of therapy. Unlike standard Reiki, the Angels are doing the attuning.

5 Component Seichem- Alex Baisley established this system in Canada. This system integrates knowingly the 5 components right into our lives in addition to prana or global life pressure to advertise recovery.

Tummo Reiki- Is thought to be the most old custom in Tibet. It integrates the real mixture of the Planet's core power (Kundalini) which is concealed in every individual with Reiki. In enhancement to recovery Tummo broadens one's devoutness as well as understanding via spiritual understanding.

Shamballa Reiki- This system assists to clean, fix as well as stabilize the physical, psychological, psychological as well as spiritual degrees of an individual. It makes use of Reiki power together with lots of vibratory signs as well as recovery rays to accomplish the function.

This recovery is much more concentrated and also specified compared to the Usui system. It is composed of 2 different attunements, 4 master signs and also 8 therapy signs. The very first sign utilized in recovery is to prepare the recipient for deep recovery as well as dealing with previous life problems.

Rainbow Reiki- Incorporates both typical and also brand-new approaches with each other to assist in a healthy and balanced state of being. In enhancement to the conventional kind of Reiki this kind additionally makes use of points for the mood, light in the Chakras, ecological formats, Crystal recovery and also mandalas, as well as exactly how to function with refined beings bodies such as quick guides). Reflection is likewise one more essential element in this kind of Reiki.

Kundalini Reiki-- Kundalini is linked with the technique of Yoga exercise. This is one of the most basic kinds of Reiki. It is launching the power from the Kundalini in this instance that advertises recovery.

In this Reiki system, the 7 Chakras produce recovery through arranging the light they originate. Rainbow Reiki is both recovery and also causes understanding of our real selves.

Imara Reiki- This Reiki is made use of to work with previous lives, quelched concerns as well as aids in far away recovery. In this Reiki, the practioner is attached to ascended masters as well as angels and also they lead the expert in their recovery procedure with the recipient.

The recipient of this kind of Reiki is needed to picture as well as practice meditation as the recovery is done to launch the power that is unfavorable so to consult. This kind of Reiki is great for kindling devoutness and also launching damaging feelings that we keep from injury as well as points of that nature.

Tummo Reiki has actually developed over the years by recognizing power readily available to us. Tummo Reiki is various from typical Reiki, it uses a very few very same approaches for recovery.

With numerous attunements, Tummo Reiki takes advantage of both Reiki as well as Kundalini to open up and also clean the Chakras. In this technique the Kundalini increases in a brief duration. Tummo is recognized with a claiming "A Course To The Heart" since it's the heart which is associated with a number of the physical body works we have actually as well as associated with recovery.

In this kind of Reiki, you are made it possible for to utilize your heart even more compared to formerly in your everyday life. Yoga exercise methods could likewise be consisted of in this kind of Reiki to open up the Kundalini.

Karuna Reiki additionally makes use of audio that is endowed with the power to recover. Karuna recovery is likewise efficient for those receivers with obsession troubles. Numerous times Karuna recovery is just utilized on those that are especially from a Karuna recovery family tree and also various other Reiki masters however it is opening up much more currently for those that require it.

Hypno Reiki- Blends both Hypnotherapies and also Reiki right into one therapy. Reiki is the recovery technique utilizing global power and also Hypnotherapy regulates the physical body as well as mind.

Reiki Aromatherapy- This is an all natural Reiki method that additionally makes use of the commercial properties of drawn out plant oils. This kind of Reiki refreshes the Mind Physical body as well as Spirit. Reiki incorporated with aromatherapy brings regarding all natural recovery impacts on the recipient.

Gendai Reki- Way Modern. Mr. Hiroshi Doi is the creator of this Reiki. He offers it a solid Buddhist viewpoint along with routine Reiki trainings.

With this type of recovery one's spiritual or spiritual idea system does not matter, it is the suggestion that all points stem from the global magnificent power, which every person could tune right into no matter of religion. This Reiki thinks simply as we require to make use of workout to maintain the physical body healthy and balanced the exact same is used to the spiritual physical body. Throughout the procedure of attunement to Spiritual Fires Reiki, your networks will certainly be progressively removed by Masters as well as Angels.

Karuna Reiki- is taken into consideration an energetic system of recovery. The words Karuna Reiki is obtained from the Sanskrit significance caring activity.

Patchouli is valued for its aphrodisiac high qualities, as well as Reiki utilizes it for dealing with allergic reactions and also skin issues. Hence, Aromatherapy in Reiki is an extra strategy to make use of the spiritual fine art of global power in a far better means.

The commercial properties in the oils could be basing, promoting, sensuous, soothing or reinforcing when made use of in combination with Reiki. It aids to create self-confidence as well as power in lengthy duration of Reiki.

Spiritual Fires Reiki- This is a spiritual recovery Reiki. The excellent point regarding this type of Reiki is there are no tough signs or methods to discover.

Below are a few other fascinating kinds of Reiki:

Gold Reiki- This Reiki system utilizes a gold ray with the life pressure power. The gold ray has numerous apartments when made use of are advantageous in Reiki recovery. This goes well with Kundalini Reiki and also one need to be a master prior to they obtain this kind of therapy.

Celtic Reiki -includes the vital force of plants as well as trees in its Reiki therapies.

Violet Fire Reiki- this type stresses recovery a pure heart devoid of ego. Understood as Quan Yin Reiki, this well-known branch of Reiki has a various means of opening up chakras as well as assisting with recovery by calling after specific global powers for their recovery. Quan Yin reintroduces us to the benefits as well as the caring power of Girl Yin and also St. Germain of the Violet Fire.

This technique could likewise be exercised in a number of various types with the usage of power tools offered in each degree of the reiki. Any person could be hip to and also utilize this approach of Reiki you do not require to have any sort of Usui training.

Huna Reiki- instructs ways to delight in life on the physical aircraft. Huna suggests secret in Hawaiian as well as this type of Reiki has actually been exercised in Hawaii for centuries. This power system puts focus on attaching to your devoutness as long as it does attaching you to the planet, your feelings, and also your physical body.

Baseding on this old custom, living a met life depends on the link as well as assimilation of your subconscious, mid uncomfortable, as well as the greater self. This practice supplies us a viewpoint of life focused in nature, mankind, love, as well as the divine. This is not simply a viewpoint; it offers us a collection of methods that are greatly transformational to a lifestyle.

Cash Stream Reiki-The Cash Stream Reiki attunement attaches you to the Creative Resource, and also assists you to clear blocks to your circulation of cash as well as earnings. Attunement in this system assists those that might have to clear blocks to their wealth, to increase their resonance to ensure that they agree with success. It opens them approximately obtain power through cash for the greatest great.

The individual sign is utilized on your own when you are experiencing economic troubles, the team sign assists recover monetary problems to those near you like friends and family and also the globe sign aids the world move their monetary situation.

Spiritual Fires Reiki- This is a spiritual recovery Reiki. Understood as Quan Yin Reiki, this recognized branch of Reiki has a various means of opening up chakras as well as aiding with recovery by calling after specific global powers for their recovery.

Cash Reiki New Fact- This Reiki kind was created in 2008 along with the monetary collapse in order to assist move some of the monetary tension individuals were experiencing. This Reiki makes use of 3 signs throughout reflection and also day-to-day recovery sessions.

Pyramid Reiki- utilizes the power of the pyramid together with the vital force of Reiki. With each other they develop a recovery resonance.

Saku Reiki - is taken into consideration a thorough kind of Reiki where the specialist makes use of a thorough system of recovery techniques. Old Egyptian Reiki- standard Reiki obtains its power from a global greater power resource; Ancient Egyptian Reiki manages this power and also transforms it right into solid recovery resonances. In enhancement to the routine concerns like all Reiki addresses crystal recovery with Reiki is likewise advantageous for kinds of psychosomatic diseases such as migraine headaches, frustrations, acid indigestion, cranky bowel disorder as well as bronchial asthma.

Wealth Success Reiki- this Reiki aids you concentrate on your economic problems and also to attain success in your life. This Reiki makes use of 2 main Hindu gods; Siren Lakshmi as well as God Ganesha.

Lakshmi is the Siren of success and also riches, both spiritual and also product. Ganesha is the God of Good luck that gives ton of money

and also success. He likewise gets rid of challenges to your product and/or spiritual objectives.

This kind of Reiki utilizes Appreciation as its major secret.

"I AM Thankfulness, I AM Wealth, I AM Success!".

This Reiki's Concept.

The Advantages of This Reiki consist of; removing those blocks (restricting ideas) which quit you from getting to wealth. It assists to link you to the doctrines of wealth, which could assist bring in and also allure cash as well as riches right into your life. Aids clear the means to materializing a partnership with cash along with clear damaging patterns around cash.

It is recommended that the 5 concepts are utilized as a book for one's life to believe concerning exactly how one's life could be boosted in the 5 locations the concepts cover. It is likewise recommended that the previously and also existing are likewise concepts that impact exactly how one believes in the minute. Reiki is a power tool for recovery so it is suggested that you assume as well as take lessons that are based on joy from your previously in order to imagine a satisfied well balanced future.

Concept 3

Simply for today, I will certainly be thankful.

Gratitude is not merely a courteous thank you to the universe. Its the understanding that simply for today every little thing you require has actually been supplied for. Individuals do not fall short to really feel appreciative when they understand they are likewise offered the present of living by Nature as well as the individuals around them.

In Reiki due to the fact that of the regulation of tourist attraction if you are thankful to just what you are enticed to it could nearly be your own. It is internal intension that is the vital component in this concept.

Chapter 5: Benefits Of Reiki Meditation

There are numerous brilliant advantages of Reiki. Reiki is a very easy procedure, yet as a rule delivers very significant impacts. The fundamental motivation behind a Reiki treatment isn't just to help the physical body, yet in addition to advance a positive personality so you can encounter more contentment throughout everyday life. The extraordinary thing about Reiki is that one doesn't need to be sick to encounter the advantages.

Some come to Reiki to help with their vitality levels, dealing with the pressure of everyday life or when changes are going on in their lives. Others use Reiki for spiritual development and experience a more prominent feeling of importance throughout everyday life. Some are well and like to remain as such, Reiki encourages them to keep up that agreement so they can react to the difficulties in an unexpected way.

After a treatment, many people would feel a lot at peace with themselves and some state that they feel vitalized, open-minded and gainful.

So many people who seek Reiki medications or Reiki training figure out that adjusting their frameworks can assist them with coping better with a wide scope of wellbeing conditions, including pressure, uneasiness, discouragement, constant torment and fruitlessness to make reference to a couple.

Advances Harmony and Balance

Reiki helps people achieve a balanced and harmonious mindset. It is a powerful, non-obtrusive energy healing methodology that improves the body's normal healthy capacity while empowering and advancing in general health. Reiki works on reestablishing harmony on all levels and works straightforwardly on the issue and condition rather than simply covering or modifying side effects.

Balance in Reiki means mental and emotional, left and right mind, male and female, marking things as fortunate or unfortunate, positive or negative and so forth.

Helps the Body to Relax

What many individuals appreciate in a Reiki treatment is that it permits them uninterrupted alone time where they aren't 'doing' but 'being'. People that have gone through a session revealed that they feel more open. Others felt a sense of serenity, and calm peace in their being.

Reiki gives the opportunity where you can be progressively mindful of what is happening inside your body and brain: To figure out how to tune in to your very own body and settle on savvy choices with respect to your prosperity from this spot. Being more aware implies that you are in your body, which causes you to access much more than inward knowing and intelligence that we, as a whole, have!

Disintegrates vitality squares and advances characteristic harmony between brain, body and soul

Customary Reiki medicines can achieve a more settled and progressively serene condition of being, where an individual is better ready to adapt to ordinary pressure. This psychological balance additionally improves learning, memory and mental clearness.

Reiki can treat mental/emotional injuries and help ease emotional swings, phobia, disappointment and even outrage. Reiki can likewise fortify and treat a person's relationship.

Since Reiki upgrades your ability to adore, it can open you up to the individuals around you and help your connections develop.

Helps the Body System to Rest

Most people spend so many resources — time and energy — in preparing for stress-responsive times. Doing this has turned into our 'standard' and our bodies truly overlook how to come back to adjust.

Reiki jogs your memory so that you can recall our bodies how to move into parasympathetic sensory system (rest/digest) self-healing mode.

Rest/think doesn't mean you need to quit being active and profitable or 'sit idle'. It enables you to rest better and reflect better which is essential to keeping up wellbeing and imperativeness. The more you are aware in this space, the more you can be active and beneficial without being pressured, depleted or burnout.

Clears the brain and improves center as you feel grounded and focused

Reiki can bolster you in remaining focused right now instead of becoming involved with laments about the past or be anxious about what's to come. It can fortify your capacity to acknowledge and work with the manner in which situations are developing in any event, when they don't follow your needs or timetable. You start to react to circumstances, individuals and yourself in a steady path as opposed to acting out of propensity.

Helps better rest

The main result of accepting a Reiki session is to relax. Whenever we're loose, we rest better, our bodies mend better, we think all the more obviously, and we identify with one another all the more truly. People will encounter profound relaxation during their Reiki session and at times a profound rest during the session also.

Quickens the body's self-mending capacity as you begin to come back to your common state

Reiki treatment rapidly returns you to your common state, or if nothing else, gets your body going the correct way.

Therefore, your breathing, pulse and circulatory system will improve as a result of the exercise. Breathing further and simpler is one of the primary things to occur during a self-practice or treatment got from another person. According to scientific researchers, when we breath better, our brain normally settles down.

As your breathing deepens, your body moves into parasympathetic sensory system (PNS) predominance for example the rest/digest stage. Your body was made to work basically in the rest/digest stage instead of the more usually experienced battle/flight stage.

Alleviates torment and supports the physical body recuperating

Outwardly looking in a Reiki treatment may give off an impression of being just a grouping of hand situations; it attempts to reestablish harmony on the most profound conceivable level. It urges your body system to improve your body's essential capacities (breathing, processing and resting) so your physical frameworks work ideally.

On the physical level, Reiki alleviates pain from headache, joint pain, sciatica, which are just some examples. It additionally assists with side effects of asthma, interminable weariness, menopausal manifestations, and sleep deprivation.

Helps profound development and passionate purifying

You don't need to be spiritual to get Reiki self-healing. However, for some, they get Reiki medications to help themselves as they heal for spiritual growth or self-development.

Reiki can make significant, regularly quick changes from within, which will result in healing the whole man and not the symptoms. For instance, it gives you direction about what to do around troublesome circumstances and this guidance will flow to you without stress. Or then again it might motivate an adjustment in the frame of mind or conviction about your circumstance. All of a sudden, you see your condition from a new point of view and can manage it in a progressively positive manner. Or then again it may guide you to the correct sort of activity required which is guided from inside.

Compliments restorative treatment and different treatments

Reiki is a brilliant compliment to regular medication as it loosens up the mind and body of patients. At the point when a patient is relaxed, the healing procedure is quickened. Individuals rest much better and are quieter after Reiki sessions.

The magnificence of Reiki is that it is non-obtrusive and is controlled in an exceptionally delicate way. The Reiki expert can give Reiki without contacting the body in situations where patients have consumed or significant wounds.

You can use Reiki safely for ailments like epilepsy, diabetes or heart conditions. You may get Reiki medications in the event that you are experiencing chemotherapy. Pregnant ladies can have Reiki medications to help them through all phases of the pregnancy.

Reiki is for everybody!

Chapter 6: Are There Safety Concerns About The Use Of Reiki?

No adverse effects were found for Reiki, due to the fact that there is nothing about a Reiki session that can interfere with conventional medical care, Reiki is unaware of contraindications and can be used with any medical procedure at the same time.

The Reiki touch is very light on or off the body. The recipient is not expected to consume any drugs, and combining substances (such as herbs) and prescription medicines are not a cause for concern.

Reiki will not override the action of medical interventions but instead support the patient through them by restoring balance to the extent possible in body, mind and spirit. Patients who feel good even when combating chronic diseases have a greater chance of completing their medical treatment and being active partners.

Because activating Reiki pulsations in the practitioner's hands settles the recipient's changing need and stops, you cannot get too much Reiki regardless of how long the hands of the practitioner remain in place.

All this said, remember that it is your responsibility to take responsibility for your own medical care and seek adequate help. Do not see your Reiki doctor for a diagnosis and do not refuse prescribed medical tests or procedures (unless he or she is also your health care provider). Call 911 in an emergency. If you are qualified in Reiki, you can securely give Reiki by putting the hand anywhere on the patient while waiting for treatment or on the way to the hospital.

Could Reiki Worsen Symptoms?

Sometimes during or after a Reiki session people experience temporary aggravation or intensification of symptoms. This could be as easy as a momentary sense of pain at the site of an ancient wound or surgical scar. This trauma is quickly resolved and can be part of the body's healing process.

Sometimes, a temporary worsening of symptoms occurs when people with chronic conditions choose to receive several (and possibly longer than usual) Reiki sessions in rapid succession.

This situation initially gives a person a better feeling of general well-being and/or relief from certain symptoms, which was followed by a brief phase in which the recipient is either very exhausted and/or returns to the symptoms. This is generally viewed as a positive response that indicates that the healing processes of the body are activated and that the brain is actively involved. A distinctive feature of this process is the fact that the client does not worry about symptoms coming back but intuits that this is just the body that does what it has to do.

The continuation of Reiki during this time provides relaxation, decreases symptoms and speeds well-being return. However, in case of doubt, whatever medical advice or health care is deemed appropriate should be sought. For example, a doctor or nurse may be able to provide guidelines and advise that no medical treatment is needed for the situation as long as this is resolved within a certain period of time.

What Does The Study Say About Reiki?

To recommend a therapy or healing practice to patients, physicians and other health practitioners need evidence that it is safe and efficient. Regarding security, no negative effects from Reiki have been reported in any of the research studies. This can be understood because no material is ingested or applied on the skin and Reiki contact is non-manipulative (and can be provided from the body if required).

Is Reiki Really Effective?

This leaves the question: does Reiki work? Or precisely, what is Reiki effective for from a research perspective?

Reiki practitioner can answer this question by saying, "Reiki is successful to restore balance and can demonstrate itself in many ways, depending on the individual's current needs." The response is not an appeal to medical researchers who use therapies for certain illnesses rather than treatments to encourage well-being or to restore balance.

Respected medical research is designed to deal with very specific issues. While a theory of homeostasis and systemic equilibrium has long been included in conventional medicine, there is traditionally no clear definition of this term which can be used to test the hypothesis that Reiki encourages balance. How would science measure the balance of an individual, given the vagueness of the term stress and the differences in the human bodies and the circumstances under which they live and operate?

Allostasis

In view of the research problem posed by the uncertainty of the word pressure, Brain Investigator Bruce McEwen of the University of Rockefeller proposed a new model using the terms allostasis. Allostasis refers to the body's attempt to protect itself from homeostasis and allostatic load refers to damage that accumulates if the attempts are managed poorly and the stress reaction is amicable.

In addition to helping people recognize the difference between beneficial and harmful stress and how to minimize this pressure, McEwen's model offers a number of steps that scientists may take to assess the impact of stress on the system and how stress can be minimized. Reiki was not practiced in this way yet.

Which findings are studied?

To date, in Reiki research primary results have used pain, anxiety and stress tests, such as blood pressure, heart rate, salivary cortisol as well as work burnout and effectiveness treatment. More detailed measures were taken to determine the effects of stroke treatment, anxiety and other chronic conditions. Provided the relatively subtle and complex nature of Reiki activities, these acts can not reflect the lived experience of Reiki recipients adequately. Measures that integrate quality of life, patient satisfaction and stress reduction will show the benefits of Reiki practice as much as possible.

What are some of the other problems in Reiki research?

Studying techniques like Reiki poses other concerns.

- Un-suitability of randomized controlled trials

Although the latest developments have shown that this research line is manipulable, randomized controlled trials are suitable for the impact of pharmaceutical products.

Yet, is the linear simplicity of the randomized controlled trial well suited for studying therapies that clearly produce complex, multilevel, rapid, and durable reactions such as Reiki? Most famous scientists don't know and there has been a debate on how best to study Reiki and other integrative treatments and therapeutic practices. Systems theory is more and more seen as a more viable way of understanding the web of integrative therapy experiences. Qualitative research can also provide a wider focus for the generation of relevant data.

Throughout Reiki science, a particular explanatory factor regulates the effects of human touch. Do the beneficiaries of Reiki have improved results because they have a positive human touch? In addition, how do you create a placebo standard for a practical technique for healing? In 1999, Reiki research introduced placebo standardization to show that participants in the studies could not differentiate between the identity of placebo and Reiki practitioners. Adding a placebo arm to Reiki research enhances the layout of the experiment and tackles the troubling human touch factor.

- Failure to track the bio-field

A further challenge to Reiki's work is the failure of contemporary technology to record, analyze and measure improvements in the biological field. Superconducting SQUIDs measure extremely small magnetic fields and can be useful for this research in the future. The rate at which technological progress is made can mean that the technology needed is on the verge of development. However, Reiki or bio-fields can also be located outside of the bio-electromagnetic spectrum.

Thankfully, science does not have to record the nature of either Reiki or the bio-field in order to measure the effect of Reiki on the human system (aspirin was used 70 years before science started to understand how it works). While certain Reiki effects, for instance an improved heart rate and blood pressure, are measurable, many commonly reported Reiki benefits, such as a sense of spiritual connection and enhanced self-esteem, cannot be quantified. These reported benefits are still important to document.

Patients who have more spiritual connection and who simply feel better may be easier to treat and more equipped to follow therapeutic protocols. This could illustrate that Reiki has an important, if indirect, effect on medical outcomes by encouraging patients ' ability to gain access to conventional medicine and a better understanding of their own needs.

What is the research status?

As the discussion on how best to study integrative therapies such as Reiki is gaining momentum, research efforts have been and continue to be conducted. Nevertheless, Reiki research has just begun. The National Institute of Health's National Center for Complementary and Integrative Health (NCCIH) completed five studies examining the ability of Reiki to benefit people with diabetes, advanced AIDS, prostate, fibromyalgia and stress.

Other published studies examined Reiki's effects on stress, blood pressure, heart rate, and immune responsiveness measurements and on subjective anxiety, pain and depression reports. Usually, the studies to date are small, and not all studies are well established. Overlapping data from a number of stronger studies however support Reiki's ability to reduce fear and pain and suggest its usefulness in inducing relaxation, improving fatigue and depressive symptoms and improving overall wellbeing. The Cochrane Systematic Review Database contains a review of the application of touch therapies for pain (including Reiki) and a protocol for Reiki use for psychological symptoms.

In order to address burnout and improve skills in healthcare and other industries and in university wellness centers, Reiki has become increasingly offered as part of wellness programs on the labor market.

Chapter 7: Animal Healer Section

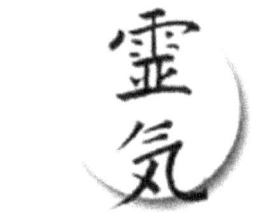

4.1 Reiki Animal Healers should heal themselves.

As a Reiki Animal Healer it is your responsibility to take care of yourself. It is your responsibility to heal yourself. You should keep in mind that the word healing and curing have different meanings. I am not implying that to be a good healer, you should be in the best health, but you should be willing to take care of yourself.

You will find in the book a section that explains the difference between healing and curing, I strongly suggest you get familiar with it.

I also invite you to start looking at animals and humans as beings made up of energy, rather then physical beings. You can still look at the physical anatomy but it is important you understand that the emotional and mental aspect of the animal is a much bigger factor that will allow it, to stay healthy and happy.

4.2 Healing vs curing

Now that you know how pets and people become sick. Let's explore the difference between healing and curing.

Curing

Curing simply means: relieving any discomfort, aches, and pains. It is also taking care of the symptoms, crises and illness. Although curing is a good thing, it can be temporary. Curing doesn't mean addressing the problem that originally created the dis-ease or dis-comfort it simply means taking care of what is a problem now, not of what started it.

By acknowledging that the root of dis-eases and dis-comfort, come from a blockage in the emotional and psychological aspects of a person, it becomes easier for us to understand that the manifestation of a dis-ease, dis-comfort, symptoms, and pain in the physical body are a mere echo of what has been happening within the persons or animals head and energy.

As a result, the blockage or stagnant energy that were originally the perpetrators, are still present or dormant within the body or energy therefore can choose at anytime to damage and put the person's health at risk.

Healing:

Healing means; going within, connecting with your heart and soul, finding the problem, releasing it and transforming the energy that once was stagnant or blocked, thus preventing the problem from reappearing, spreading further or creating any additional problems.

Healing also means: Reconnecting the body and soul so that they may work in harmony with one another, thus creating and maintaining good health in the mind, body and spirit.

Healing can also be described as: a self empowering journey that allows the person suffering from the illness to take the precaution needed in order to regain a healthy body by restructuring her or his inner and outer dialogue, reprogramming his own brain with beliefs that build him up rather then limit him, and to adjust his perception about himself, other people, life and events.

Healing begins when awareness takes place and ends with positive transformations. Healing takes time, no medication can bring you to that state of being, but going within will.

4.3 The Animal Reiki Practitioner Code of Ethics

Animal Reiki Practitioners are expected to conform to a code of ethic and to abide by it under all circumstances. The ethical code focuses upon the relationship developed and maintained between the practitioner and the animals he treats.

Animal Reiki Practitioner vow to:

☐ I recognize the animals as being equal partners on this planet. Therefore they have the same rights as I do.

☐ I respect and honor the animal kingdom.

☐ I honor and respect the lessons taught by the animals.

☐ acknowledge that giving a Reiki treatment to an animal is a gift of compassion and love. I therefore vow to serve as a channel of pure and unconditional love.

☐ I nurture the relationship between the animals and I.

☐ I am grateful for the opportunity I have received to help and heal the animal kingdom.

☐ I develop and maintain a loving and respectful relationship with the animal kingdom.

☐ I work in partnership with the animals.

☐ I always ask the animal permission before giving them a Reiki healing session.

☐ I accept and respect the animal decision.

☐ I observe the animal body language, and listen carefully at all time for the messages the animal is giving me.

☐ I put aside my ego, I open up my heart and channel the energy needed to treat the animals.

☐ I put my expectations aside and remain neutral throughout the entire healing process.

☐ I recognize that the healing offered to the animal is not about my own personal abilities but rather about the animal own healing journey.

☐ I let go of all expectation and let creator do his work.

☐ I accept the results and give gratitude for the result received during the Reiki healing session.

For the Healer:

☐ I vow to take care of myself.

☐ I vow to feed myself well.

☐ I vow to love and honor myself.

☐ I vow to let go of my ego.

☐ I vow to heal myself when needed.

☐ I vow to let go of judgment.

☐ I vow to have a positive perception.

☐ I vow to nourish to release any negative emotions, thoughts and pattern that may alt my spiritual and intuitive awakening.

Chapter 8: Meditation In Preparation For Healing

When Dr. Usui developed his reiki healing practice, he highlighted 5 different principles to guide his learners towards achieving the proper healing technique. These principles come together to form *Hatsurei-Ho* - otherwise known as reiki guided meditation. The purpose of the practice is to focus the healers mind and to open their body to the positive impact that reiki can have on their life force.

Before starting off any reiki healing session - whether on yourself or on anyone else - it's important to start with guided meditation first. This removes any impurities from your energy, improving the flow of your life force and heightening positive energy for a more enriching, effective healing experience.

21st Thing you need to know…

Understanding the Phrasing for Reiki Principles

One thing you'll notice about each reiki meditation principle is that they're all preceded by the phrase "just for today." Before you engage in meditation, it's important to understand **why that specific phrase is an important part of the entire principle.**

There are lots of meditation practices out there that encourage you to formulate impossible promises to yourself and to others around you, that might not actually be doable. In effect, you feel guilty and unhappy when you fail to meet the promises you made during your meditation practice.

That's why the reiki healing meditation practice encourages you to start each principle with *"just for today."* The practice understands that not everyone can experience a flawless flow of energy every day for their entire lives. Disturbances to your life force - whether in the form of illness or emotional baggage or anything in between - can and will happen somewhere down the line.

The objective of the reiki meditation practice is not to pressure you into adhering to your promises or to formulate unrealistic goals that you might not reach. Instead, it understands that guidance and healing is something that we all need *on a daily basis*. So, if for some reason, you find that today doesn't work out in your favor, there will always be tomorrow.

Once you're able to fully understand the way that these principles are phrased, then you can experience the complete benefits of the guided meditation practice.

22nd Thing you need to know…

Just for Today, I Will Not Worry

The first principle in the reiki meditation practice is *"just for today, I will not worry."* As the first principle, it does hold significant importance compared to some of the others on the list. The basic idea is that **_worry_** uses your positive energy and converts it to negativity. When you spend your time thinking too much about future events, you'll find that it will impact your entire life negatively.

Instead of focusing on negativities and worrying about things that you can't completely predict, approach situations with a positive, can-do attitude. Assess what you're worrying about. Can you change it? Can you do something about it? If you answered yes, then that's precisely what you should do. If you answered no, then there's no need to worry.

23rd Thing you need to know...

Just for Today, I Will Not Be Angry

Anger is one of the strongest emotions people feel. And as you would have expected, it's also responsible for a lot of the stress and negativity we feel. While anger is an appropriate response to a variety of situations, there is a limit as to the extent of anger that's healthy for *you*.

If you allow anger to transform your energy and limit your positivity, you will experience its negative impacts on your life force. What's more, anger that's not resolved will come back in uglier ways later on. That's why it's important to make sure that you avoid anger at all costs.

The second principle of the reiki meditation process encourages practitioners to refuse anger. There are better, more tactful ways to address frustrating situations. Be one step ahead of yourself at all times and make a firm resolve to refuse the negative impact of anger on your wellness.

Remember - your objective isn't to preserve the feelings of the person who wronged you, but to preserve your own positive energy.

24th Thing you need to know...

Just for Today, I Will Do My Work Honestly

You are naturally gifted and talented, with abilities that are beneficial not only to yourself, but to others around you. When you perform your work with the basic intention of just 'getting it over with', you cheat others and yourself because you're capable of much, much more.

As the third principle for reiki meditation, the goal of doing your work honestly is to perform your tasks **to the best of your abilities** and not just because you want to get them done. Offer up your best and be honest in all that you do - you'll give justice to your natural talents and gifts, and enrich your energy and life force along the way.

25th Thing you need to know...

Just for Today, I Will Be Thankful for My Blessings

When was the last time you took a step back to look at all the different ways that you've been blessed? All too often, we focus on the negative things in our lives. Plans that don't go our way, overdue bills, angry bosses and difficult coworkers - it's easy to see all the different aspects of our lives that might not be what we want them to.

But maintaining your attention on these negative events can cause bad energy to thrive in your system. The foundation of a positive outlook is an awareness of the many wonderful blessings that you have in your life. The more readily you're able to pick out these blessings, the stronger your positivity becomes.

26th Thing you need to know…

Just for Today, I Will Be Kind to My Neighbor and All Living Things

These days, it's easy to lose track of all the other living creatures around us. As the 'selfie' generation, we tend to put ourselves as the center of our lives, creating a negative, 'every-man-for-himself' mentality. But the change starts with you.

As part of your meditation practice, keep your neighbor and the other wonderful creatures of the world in mind. Acknowledge that their experiences are real and valid, and that they are equally as important as you are. The more you value the lives of others around you, the easier it becomes for you to appreciate anything and everything that happens around you.

27th Thing you need to know…

Hasturei-Ho Follows a Process

The Hatsurei-Ho practice follows a specific, guided process in order to help healers cleanse their energy and prepare for the reiki healing technique. By following this structured method, you open up the opportunity to perform reiki healing with optimized life force flowing through your system.

28th Thing you need to know…

The First Step: Seiza

Start off in a comfortable seated position with the legs tucked under the body. An alternative pose would be to sit up straight in a chair.

29th Thing you need to know...

The Second Step: Mokuken

In a state of mindfulness, mention the intention "I'm beginning Hatsurie-Ho." During this time, you can start meditating on the five principles mentioned above. Keep in mind that your objective is to *cleanse your life force*.

30th Thing you need to know...

The Third Step: Kenyoku

At this point, you will start the process of dry bathing. The objective of this step is to cleanse the body and remove any impurities by using the clean, positive energy around you.

Position your right hand over your left shoulder, and then swipe diagonally downwards. Do the same with your opposite hand and shoulder.

Open your right palm and extend your arm. Your hand should be parallel with the floor, with your palm facing upwards.

Position your left hand over your right shoulder and move your hand over the length of your right arm towards your open palm. Envision the negativity in your system being swept away and collected into your palm during the process.

Repeat the previous step using your opposite hand and arm.

31st Thing you need to know…

The Fourth Step: Joshin Kokyu Ho

This breathing technique spreads positive life force throughout your body. Breathe in deeply through your nose, and visualize the energy flowing through your nostrils all the way to your root chakra. Exhale out involving your entire being in the process. Repeat the breathing slowly and deliberately for at least 10 minutes, aiming to live in the ***now***.

32nd Thing you need to know…

The Fifth Step: Gassho

During this phase, your objective is to localize your energy into a single focal point. Press your palms together and focus on your middle fingers. Breathe in and out gently and deliberately and visualize the energy mounting where your middle fingers are pressed together.

33rd Thing you need to know...

The Sixth Step: Seishin Toitsu

Visualize the energy in your middle fingers moving to your root chakra each time you exhale. When you inhale, visualize the energy moving back into your fingertips. Avoid tracing the energy moving through your arms, your chest, and then down to your root chakra. Instead, focus on visualizing the energy passing immediately to the root chakra from your fingers and back again with each inhale and exhale. Perform this for about 5 minutes.

34th Thing you need to know...

The Seventh Step: Mokunen

Once the meditation is over and you feel calm and cleansed, then utter the words "I am now ending Hatsurei Ho." to seal the practice.

Keep in mind that this process of cleansing your energy and meditating isn't only beneficial in preparation for reiki healing. Finding time for this meditation process even when you don't intend to perform any healing can help keep your energy positive, and will help you maintain optimal wellness to prevent pent up negativity from building up inside your system.

35th Thing you need to know...

Refocus With Your Intention

As you go through the process of meditation, it would help to maintain or regain focus by reminding yourself of your intention. Repeat the intention to yourself like a mantra every so often to help keep your mind on the goal of your reiki healing session. If you have to, don't be afraid to word it out. Often, hearing the intention come from your own lips helps make it much more prominent in your mind.

36th Thing you need to know…

Activate Reiki Energy

During the meditation process, you should have been able to activate the reiki energy within yourself. If you feel like you need to heighten the energy even more, then you may need to follow a few more steps before you begin.

Hold your hands up to the sky with your palms facing upwards. Breathe deeply for a few minutes until you achieve a state of calm mindfulness. Visualize the positive ideas and feelings in your crown as an intense glow of bright, white light. Feel this energy travel down your head to your shoulders, arms, and finally to your hands.

Bring your hands slowly downwards and make them face each other, palm to palm, almost touching. Feel the warmth of the bright white healing energy as it grows between your palms. Hold the position for a few moments until you feel it's strong enough for healing.

Chapter 9: Individual Elements

Water: The Water element is reflected in the energy of winter. It is the essence of your will power, and the potential of manifestation in your life. Your ability to draw vitality from your life essence is a primary focus of the water element. The Water element meridians are the Bladder and Kidney meridians. Water is gentle when in balance, and fearful when not in balance.

Wood: The Wood element is reflected in the energy of spring, and empowers your vision and perspective to project the planning necessary for your life goals. Your wood element gives you growth, stability, creativity, and flexibility to move ahead with your life. The wood element is also a catalyst for your healing. The Liver & Gall Bladder meridians are of the Wood element. Wood is kind when in balance, and angry when not in balance.

Fire: The Fire element is reflected in the energy of summer, and it helps you to mature by energetically embracing your life in a joyful and passionate way. It facilitates your connectedness from the heart in all kinds of relationships. The Heart, Small Intestine, Pericardium and Sanjiao (AKA triple burner)meridians are of the Fire element. Fire is joyful when in balance, and raging when out of balance.

Earth: The Earth element is reflected in the energy of late summer. It is the seat of your intention. This energy enables you to nurture, accept, and support others for the sake of service. It helps you to feel the pain and suffering of others with compassion and thoughtfulness. It assists you in your stability and grounding, so that you can support yourself and others through right action. The Spleen & Stomach meridians are of the Earth element. Earth is satisfied when in balance, and worried when out of balance.Earth element brings stability, strength, comfort and grounding. The person who has balanced their earth element can feel a deep connection with the earth and feel more rooted or grounded. These people are able to be calm and have better thoughts and also can balance their lives. This helps to make sure the energy flows and it removes all the blockages created during the different phases of life. The blockages are created mainly due to greediness, laziness, attention seeking attitude, narrow-minded thoughts and overly materialistic gain thoughts.

Metal: The Metal element is reflected in the energy of autumn. It helps you to let go of attachments on all levels of your being. The metal element helps you to separate the pure from the impure in your world, and to determine your standards. The metal element also connects you to spirit, enables you to "believe", and find meaning and purpose in your life. The emotion of Metal is Grief. The Lung &

Large Intestine meridians are of the Metal element. Metal is courageous when in balance, and depressed when out of balance.

Crystals for Reiki

Crystals have been used for centuries as tools for healing and increasing levels of awareness with each stone being specially selected for specific frequencies and properties. Although combining Reiki with the use of crystals is relatively new, this branch of Reiki has the potential to not only transform your current Reiki practice, but our world as well.

Crystal Reiki utilizes the frequencies that reside within the earth and amplifies them through the power of Reiki energy. By infusing these powerful vibrations with the consciousness of Reiki energy, the shifts can be targeted and profound.

The earth vibrates at a specific frequency known as the Schumann resonance. Traditionally this resonance is thought to hover around 7.8 Hz though it varies from region to region. Since 1980's however this frequency has been thought to be rising. This is interesting because science is beginning to understand that we are impacted deeply by the earth's resonance and as it increases, the dissonance between our own frequency and that of the earth is felt deeply on all levels.

These frequencies are thought to impact our autonomic nervous system, brain and cardiovascular system.In your life and the world around you, you may be noticing that things are getting more polarized.

People are gravitating towards the ends of the spectrum with regard to emotions and consciousness. As the frequency of our planet increases, we are given a choice to either raise our own awareness and frequency so that we will feel resonance with earth or to resist it and feel the effects of physical imbalance as well as mental/emotional chaos.

These shifts in the earth's geomagnetic activity are correlated with hospital admissions, death from heart attacks and strokes, as well as many other physical imbalances such as depression, fatigue, mental confusion, and even the number of traffic accidents that occur.

Our body's ability to maintain balance is greatly impacted by the shifts in frequency of the earth. Studies have even connected major political and social events to the earth's energetic activity such as solar flares.

In one study, 80% of the most significant events occurred when solar activity was at its peak. On the flip side, it is thought that just as the frequencies of the earth impact us, our collective frequencies also have a dramatic effect on our planet. There have been studies that show when a group of individuals unite in a state of awareness, the randomness in their environment is reduced.

A study that examined the ability of an individual to affect the DNA was conducted by cellular biologist Glen Rein. The individual's studied were trained to elicit specific emotions such as love and appreciation and then hold a test tube of DNA.

When tested, there was no significant change in the test tube samples. Rein then had a second group of trained individuals create not only the positive emotions, but also hold an intention which in this study was to either wind or unwind the strands of DNA in the sample they were holding. In this group there were significant changes in the DNA with some samples being wound or unwound as much as 25%. The third group of participants were asked to hold only the intention without a positive emotional state and the samples with this group experienced no change.

In this study, the combination of the intention of the practitioner with their own state of presence elicited significant change. Just as thought needs the catalyst of presence to be effective, crystals need the energetic infusion of universal life force to transmit their balancing properties.

The combination of Reiki and the crystals you use will create a unique electromagnetic signature that will send a specific signal out into the field and draw in the information needed to fulfill the set intentions. Crystal Reiki has the potential to connect you with the rising consciousness around you and help you align with it and use it to help yourself and others. As we connect and in a state of presence use Reiki energy to amplify the energy of the crystals we work with, that energy can in turn positively impact the earth so that a symbiotic relationship can be created.

One study demonstrated that even a group of 2,500 individuals taking time to be present through meditation elicited a

25% reduction in crime rates in a population of one and a half million.

In your Crystal Reiki sessions you will not only be in a state of heightened awareness, but you will be harnessing the universal life force energy and using crystals to focus and refine that frequency. As Aristotle noted, the whole is greater than the sum of its parts. Together, within the specific energy field of our work, miracles can occur with the individuals we work with and with our world.

How Crystals for Reiki works

In a Crystal Reiki session, you will use specifically selected crystals and place them in a specific layout around and on the recipient and then allow Reiki energy to flow through you into the crystals and then the recipient. Just as sunlight shining through a crystal prism creates facets of light, Reiki energy passing through the crystals will create a specific energetic resonance within the recipient that their body will then use to address specific imbalances.The presence of Reiki energy amplifies the energy of the crystals and helps the bodymind of the recipient focus on specific areas of the body, conditions or levels of awareness that are ready to heal. In a Crystal Reiki session, Reiki energy is coming from above through the crown chakra while the crystals used in the session bring in a grounding energy from the earth. Together these energies work seamlessly. Crystals are solid symmetrical structures with regularly ordered atoms and molecules that are packed in repeating patterns which extend in all three dimensions of space. The shape and atomic structure of a crystal define it. The defects within a crystal can also define its healing properties and rather than being seen as irregularities, can be intuitively used with powerful effects. Although crystals are considered a part of the mineral kingdom, minerals are less transparent than crystals and darker in color with a consistent chemical structure. Minerals are thought to strengthen the physical aspects of the body such as bones, tissue etc. Both minerals and crystals can be used to help balance the recipient in a Crystal Reiki session. Similarities can be found in the structures of a crystal and our own DNA with dodecahedrons and icosahedrons found in both.The healing properties of each crystal can be associated with the way in which it was formed. Much of the earth's crystals were formed millions of years ago. Crystals are formed in liquid such as magma or water as well as gas that is pushed up from the earth. As the liquid evaporates, the minerals within that liquid bond. The harder crystals are formed within higher temperatures.The geopathic stress that is present as a crystal is formed also has an impact on its healing properties, with enhanced properties present. You will find that the same type of crystal found in different areas with different geopathic stresses will hold different resonances. Regardless of form, crystals have the ability to absorb, channel, focus and emit energy. The energy of Reiki will infuse the intentions of the practitioner and recipient as well as the energetic properties of the crystal to create a unique high frequency.

Crystals can generate energy through a process known as the Piezoelectric effect. This effect occurs when pressure is applied to the crystal which then generates energy. In the same way, if a voltage is applied to a crystal such as quartz, it will bend or slightly change its shape. We all consist of electromagnetic energy. When holding a crystal, your frequency interacts with the crystal, creating a similar type of Piezoelectric effect. The crystal vibrates and the energy it creates can be transmitted to your own internal energy pathways. One key factor that separates Crystal Reiki from general Crystal Healing is the foundational principles of Reiki.

As Reiki practitioners, we understand that our role is to be the observer that holds space for the healing within the recipient to occur. We do not diagnose or prescribe and allow the recipient's body to be the active participant in their healing.

We are also detached from the outcome. Although we set intentions at the start of a Crystal Reiki session and use our intuition as well as our understanding of crystals to focus the energy of the session, we understand that the session will proceed exactly as the recipient's body needs it to and for the highest good of all concerned.

With no expectations, we also do not use our own personal energy in the session. Crystal Reiki sessions instead are an energizing and healing experience for both the recipient and practitioner because Reiki energy is the amplifier in the session. Continued work with Crystal Reiki helps the practitioner to raise and balance their own awareness which extends to all areas of their life and helps to be a healing force in the lives of everyone they touch.

A Crystal Reiki practitioner uses Reiki energy to create a state of presence that is focused and accesses a higher level of consciousness. This presence holds the space for Reiki energy to activate and amplify the crystal energy for a specific purpose so that the desired outcome can be achieved.

Chapter 10: Exciting Times

Many people train in level one and decide that is all they need. Those who go on to level two sometimes want to be able to treat members of the public and be paid for this. When I did level two, I just felt the need to use the energy for myself and my family. I never thought I would want to take it any further and for the next two years I was content with this. Then the synchronicity continued. I had been visiting a crystal shop for a couple of years and the couple running it decided to take over the shop next door and make it into a therapy room. It had been a dream of theirs for years. As many therapists over the years had visited and left business cards with them, they had got to know them all well. They made the decision to ask five or six therapists that they gelled with to work in the therapy shop and I was chosen to be one of them at weekends, so I could continue my day job. The therapy shop was filled with billowing sales from the ceiling and lovely ambient lighting, including a lovely colour changing light which I now have in my therapy room. Until this point, I had never thought of using reiki outside the circle of family and friends. This was my next learning curve.

My new therapy space came about as I used my home for foreign language students to stay with me all year round. One day I was complaining to one of the shop owners that I had no "me" space anymore as all my rooms were taken. He mentioned my attic and I gave him the sad story. He advised me once my attic was fixed to let him know and he would build a corner of it into a space for me to meditate. When I advised him months later that it was now sorted, he spent a few days in my attic and said I was not allowed to look. He then took me shopping for some wood panelling. When it was finished, I absolutely loved it. He not only gave me a meditation space, he also converted the whole attic into a wonderful space for me. The atmosphere in it is wonderful, plus his wife made me an Angel from feathers to hang from my window and my Son in law made me a Fairy Door for it too. I was later, after becoming more comfortable, able to use it for clients as well.

Soon after this I had a spiritual reading from my teacher David and was advised that he saw I had a spare room in my house and was seen to be treating people sitting on a chair. He did not know if this was friends or clients. At the time I was not comfortable treating strangers in my home. After a while I decided to think about it and determined to get myself a therapy bed for the room even though

David had not seen a bed. On checking out prices I thought I would not be able to afford one. That Christmas an aunt gave me unexpected money for Christmas by doubling what she had previously given me, and I then saw brand new Therapy beds on eBay for auction and managed to get one for the money I now had. Initially this was used to have exchange visits with my friend and other therapists. It was not until later that it was opened to the public. I have since found that often, all I need do is put a thought out there and it materialises in time.

Since then I have never looked back and love treating clients in my home. Often, I will chat for quite a bit after the therapy session. I feel gratitude that I do not make all my living from reiki. This means I do not have back to back clients and can enjoy their company after the therapy session if required. It never ceases to amaze me how much reiki helps people and often people want to talk more in depth about it. Sometimes they decide to learn to do it themselves and the next time I see them it can be for a reiki workshop.

Crystals

Now with my work in the therapy shop I was introduced to all sorts of crystals and found out some fascinating things. While I had been in a bad marriage, I had been drawn to collecting jewellery all made of Hematite. At that time, I just thought it was pretty. I never even knew it was a crystal. I found out that this is a grounding and protecting crystal. The interesting thing is when my marriage came to an end the pieces of jewellery starting breaking or one half of a pair of earrings would mysteriously disappear. I now no longer needed the protection of the hematite and was happy to explore other crystals to wear and built up a lovely collection of all colours which I could use depending on my mood or need. Another interesting thing that happens with the crystal Amber, is I cannot keep it. Any jewellery that I get given decides to remove itself from me. I always remember a friend giving me a beautiful Amber pendant. The first time I wore it to work, by the time I had got there it had fallen off on the way. This was the last time I ever used Amber. Interestingly I found out that the crystal has the following properties.

I had got rid of the negative energy, had no headaches, was calm and patient. You get my meaning, I didn't need this crystal in my life.

Balances emotions.

Attracts good luck.

Eliminates fears.

Relieves a headache.

Clears the mind.

Dissolves negative energy.

Helps develop patience and wisdom.

One incident that took place in the therapy shop was me going in to treat a client. As I stood over the therapy table, I felt sick and believed I was being pulled over. On looking underneath, one of the other therapists had left a large ball of Obsidian which is a grounding stone. After that, we made sure that all crystals were removed once someone had finished with a client! Crystals can have super strong energy.

I decided to explore more about crystals and the first book I bought was The Crystal Bible by Judy hall. This explains crystals in an informative way. You can look under properties or colours. It's often my first "go to" book when I am trying to find the right crystal to use for anything. I then went on to read more of her books which include more "New Age" crystals. Crystals are really nothing new as the Egyptians used them too.

This then led me to want to learn more about using crystals for our health and I heard about a crystal course so decided to sign up for it. Before I went on the course,

I decide to visit a crystal therapist. At that stage I had no idea what was to take place. I certainly got a surprise but think that synchronicity once again played out. I was a member of a metaphysical group. This was a group where we talked about many interesting subjects including ghosts and out of body experiences as well as reiki and meditation. The person running it had relocated to Edinburgh, and as she had set one up in her last city decided it was our time. Guess what she was? That's right - she was a crystal therapist!

The crystal therapist I visited had a selection of very big crystals in the room and gave me some interesting information about them. One was a massive Smokey Quartz and as it was used over time, was becoming clearer and clearer. It was the first time I had been aware that could happen. She also had crystals that were record keepers and she advised me they all had a story to tell. She told me a story of taking a client into another room to put his hands on a large quartz crystal. Just as she left him there holding the crystal the doorbell rang. She ended up having a long conversation on the door step- approximately forty minutes, totally forgetting about her client! When she returned to the room to apologise to the client, he replied that he thought only five minutes had passed. The power of crystals can be amazing.

I lay down not knowing what to expect as she gave me a crystal to hold and placed others around me. At this point I was very surprised to find out that she was also clairvoyant. She started giving me information about my past life while treating me during the therapy hour. Funnily enough It all made sense to me. I was also buzzing with the energy of the crystals she used on and around me. I was now looking forward to the crystal course even more.

During the Melody Crystal course one of the things we were taught was past life ascension which takes you back in time for you to find information to help you today. This is not the same as past life regression as the emotions do not become involved. Guess where I went? I was back to the situation the crystal therapist had spoken to me about. I remember saying I did not want to do the same things as I had done in the past which was taking care of a sick mistress. I then realised at this point, many people that come to me for therapy have various health issues, so in a way I am continuing in the same vein. The only difference now is I have a life outside my clients. Even though I love working with reiki clients, a good work / life balance is important.

When I went home after the course finished, my head was full of information for me to practise so I started with friends and family. My experience with my daughter was amazing and gave us both a lot to discuss. I am sure most mothers do not get opportunities like this with their children, but this was only the beginning. The interesting part of this was she saw someone reading a book but could not work out what it was. After spending a few minutes, she was able to see it was a book that I had given her to read about reiki. She said that was her reminder to get reading it.

I was blown away but how much I learned in such a short time, about all the ways you can use crystals to change your life, and even get information from the past. I also wanted to learn more about the basics of the different types of crystals and what they could be used for. Around this time my daughter became pregnant. My friend Anne had started to use Pendulums and asked if my daughter would give permission to try and learn the sex of the baby. We were all excited to see the outcome. When Anne asked it was a girl the pendulum moved in a way to indicate "no". When asked about a boy it started swinging wildly in the other direction. I asked if I could try and went through the same questions, but I did not get the same answers. It answered "can't decide" to both questions from me. I then changed the question and asked if it was going to give me an answer. At this point it went very strongly in the "no" direction. It seems that as grandmother to be it decided I should wait for the birth to find out if I was going to have a grandson or granddaughter!

Soon after this, my reiki teacher was holding a crystal workshop, and it was here that I was introduced to using a crystal pendulum properly. He had hidden things in his garden such as bottles of essential oils and we had to find them by asking the pendulum to give a sign for yes and no. Sure enough after asking things such as "Is it in this area?" and getting a "no" answer I would move on by asking more questions and was finally taken to see my crystal that I was to find halfway up a tree. I remember to this day David coming up to me as I was standing looking silly. He asked me if I had a problem. I advised the crystal pendulum had said my item was not to the left or right of where I was standing. Apparently, it was exactly where I was now, but I could not see it. He advised me to look up and sure enough my bottle of essential oils was up in a tree directly above my head. What a fun day that was.

As all energy vibrates at different frequencies, reiki and crystals are no different, and I often use them together when I am treating clients. I sometimes use pendulums to check if people's Chakras (energy points) need a little attention. I then use one to check which the correct crystals to use are. It's amazing how I will be told no, no, then yes as I lay my hands on the right crystal for my clients. These can all then help rebalance the body. One of my favourite crystals is Blue lace agate which can help with communication. It's great if you must stand in front of a lot of people or need to have an awkward conversation with someone. I remember a teacher telling me she always carried a piece as she did a lot of talking to adults. When another teacher asked for help with a discussion she needed to lead, the other let her borrow her crystal. The second teacher felt confident enough to go on and do her talk.

Many crystals have specific properties to help with problems. These may be depression, infertility, nightmares, grounding- the list goes on and on. As I mentioned, my first crystal book was The Crystal Bible by Judy Hall. To this day it is one that I use the most. Funny enough when I was looking for names for my two new puppies a few years later I thought of Merlin for the male. The next day I picked up the Crystal Bible and saw that months before I even thought of getting puppies, I had placed a piece of paper in the page for Merlinite. It was obviously the correct name for him.

Through my love of crystals, I introduced one of my grandsons to them. I remember the first time he visited the crystal shop and was given enough money to buy two crystals. He bought two of the same which were Amethyst. The shop owner told him to pick another two for free, so he chose two Blue Lace Agate. I found this interesting as I thought he would have picked four different crystals. When we got back to my home, he kept transferring the agate from one hand to another and we chatted. My daughter advised he had a problem the previous night when he was meant to talk to his father over the phone. He had advised he wanted to talk but couldn't. Funnily enough Blue Lace Agate helps communication problems and that evening he was then able to speak to his father. I was then advised he had been suffering nightmares. Once again, he had chosen the correct crystal in Amethyst. This is the same grandson that wanted to train in reiki. I think he has a real affinity with crystals and energy. He now has a collection of crystals both from me and those he has bought himself. He loves the crystals so much that he has acquired all his mother's crystals as well. His younger sister also now collects crystals although she does not have as big an interest in them. It's interesting that from having reiki in the womb and loving crystals he went on to also train in reiki.

Even though reiki helped me kill the pain in my back it did not stop it going into crisis for the simplest thing. My back was a problem for me as I could not do many things in my life and I was always frightened that my back would go again by doing the simplest thing. A short time before it went again, someone had introduced me to the Sun Ancon Chi Machine.

Chapter 11: Reiki & Stress Relief

During childbirth, we bring into this life, a supply of Kid/chi vitality to fuel the body's nature healing capabilities. When we can't replenish that vitality for a delayed period, we might become physically or candidly sick. Pressure/stress not discharged is put away in the filaments of the body's organs, muscles, and connective tissue. Over time, this put away strain becomes a lethal type of strength, blocking the stream of this vitality through the body, and in addition the body's ability to ingest it, in the long run causing any of the preventable diseases experienced in the Western World.

A Reiki treatment furnishes the beneficiary with a concentrated, capable infusion/booster shot of this life power/Reiki vitality, and parities its stream and assimilation in the body. The practitioner providing the therapy goes about as a channel or conduit for the concentrated stream of this vitality from the practitioner's hands into the beneficiary's body. The beneficiary, then, applies that vitality however, and where ever it is required. No individual vitality is drawn from the practitioner. Unexpectedly, the practitioner is all the while revived and strengthened.

Training to be a Reiki Channel/practitioner is directed in three stages/attunements. The primary degree (Level 1) gives the practitioner the tools for self healing. The second degree (Level 2) gives the tools to bolster others in their healing endeavors.

The Origins of Reiki:

This natural healing system is described in 2,500-year old Sanskrit writings. That places its practice at about 600 years BCE, in the India-Tibet range. That would be within 100 years or so of when Lao Tzu is said to have written or coordinated the writing of the Tao Te Chin. Nobody knows how old the practice really is.

In the nineteenth century, a Japanese friar or school professor (depending on who you read), Dr. Mikado Usual, rediscovered the practice as an aftereffect of his own 20-year journey to take in the basis for the act of healing with the hands. Dr. Mikado is said to have taken the practice back to Japan, where he continued to educate and rehearse the procedure for the remainder of his life. This "Usual system" of vitality healing has since been gone around Reiki Masters, and is presently drilled on an overall basis.

Dr. Usual coined the Japanese expression, Reiki, which portrays this healing procedure. Reiki is really two words, or characters in kanji. The character, Reid, portrays the grandiose, widespread part of the vitality being referred to, and the character, kid, speaks to the major life drive that streams normally through all things.

How Reiki Affects Your Body:

The body has its own nature healing capabilities that are energized by this widespread life/Reiki vitality. Reiki therapy replenishes the beneficiary's Reiki vitality supply, while removing blockages to the vitality stream, and balancing its ingestion by every last cell of the body. During this procedure, the beneficiary moves into a profound condition of unwinding, softening and relaxing every muscle, connective tissue, and organ in the body. That softening evacuates the blockages of vitality stream and makes all filaments and cells in the body spongier to the Reiki vitality and supplements ingested and breathed.

The body extends its capacity to breath. The heart rate drops. More successful oxygen move results in a more noteworthy quantity of oxygen being conveyed to the brain and in addition every other organ in the body. The body's metabolism works simply like every other burning framework. The more oxygen is conveyed the more compelling the procedure. Thinking becomes clearer. Insights into specific inquiries or issues happen all the more promptly. The normal chemicals created by the body become those connected with resisting infection and disease, instead of those that backing the battle/flight situation, for example, the stress hormone, adrenaline.

The Benefits and/or Drawbacks of Reiki:

An ordinary Reiki treatment takes around 60 minutes. Notwithstanding a stressful occasion or situation, however, a level 1 practitioner can decrease the body's creation of the stress hormone, adrenaline, in only a couple of minutes, by placing the hands over the kidneys – that is extremely close to the adrenal gland that delivers that hormone when conditions become stressful.

At the point when that mindfulness happens, releasing the pressure is as simple and brisk as a profound moan with the hands set over the heart, the sternum, or the kidneys.

Practitioners giving treatment experience the same rejuvenating energize as is experienced by the beneficiary often leaving the treatment with the same feelings of peace and well-being.

Self healing is a significant initial step to becoming a channel for Reiki vitality. Just when you have assumed liability for your own particular health and well-being would you be able to position yourself to assist others in their own healing procedures. Self treatment diminishes stress, unwinds you, and strengthens your energy to resist sickness. At a more elevated amount, it also brings amicability and well-being into your life.

How does reiki can relief you pain:

Reiki has turned out to be an exceptionally powerful pain and stress management tool for me over the past three years. The real incident that Reiki assisted me with was because of an auto crash where I was back finished at a stop-sign, the other auto was traveling at around 30 mph and slammed my vehicle into the auto in front (also stationary). Luckily, there were no broken bones, just soft tissue harm. However, because of having von Will brand Disease, I (in the same way as other of you) couldn't take the calming prescriptions to help with recovery and because of my own sensitivity to pain solution, was relying on Tylenol versus more grounded analgesics.

The whiplash from the mishap required active recuperation. The scope of movement enhanced over two or three months of PT however the pain was still intense, so I looked for the assistance of Dana Young, an expert Reiki practitioner. The main session yielded recognizable pain help and power unwinding, the following sessions continued to diminish the pain and increase the time between the fits. After two years, I have what the orthopedic specialists would call an interminable neck pain. Once in a while I'll take Tylenol to facilitate the pain if a fit goes ahead, however I realize that a Reiki session will dependably be more powerful long haul; helping my body to mend rather than cover manifestations.

The following is a portrayal of Reiki from the Master Reiki Practitioner that I've seen for the past 3 years, Dana Young of Dragonfly Reiki:

Reiki is a relaxing light touch therapy that assists the mind and body in returning to its common condition of parity. Clinical perception and some preliminary confirmation from little studies show that Reiki treatment can be gainful for:

- stress mitigation
- Anxiety and sadness
- Pain, discomfort and other palliative consideration
- Insomnia
- Digestive issues

- improved heart rate variables in cardiovascular patients
- Side impacts from tumor treatment, including queasiness and exhaustion
- Recovery from surgery or games injury
- Overall well-being.

Definitive benefits connected with Reiki treatment are to feel healthier and more content and advance toward a condition of more prominent mindfulness. These ideas are like other types of Eastern-based medicine and mind/body works on, including meditation, Tai Chi, I Gong, yoga, acupuncture, Traditional Chinese Medicine and shiatsu.

Reiki is anything but difficult to learn as a practice for self-care and adjust. Self-treatment is particularly useful for people undergoing treatment for health issues, or who live with nonstop health conditions.

Reiki treatment is a strong tool for use as a supplement to customary medicine, and is increasingly being offered in numerous hospitals, restorative consideration and therapeutic settings. Reiki treatment ought not to be a substitute for general therapeutic consideration from a qualified professional.

As a physically dynamic individual, my body is pushed really hard. With the riskier sports like snowboarding where a fall could prompt terrible bruising or broken bones, I take insurances by using Humane-P beforehand (and obviously wear a head protector!). However, if an injury is a sprain, muscle pull or other type of harm that may take more time to recuperate, I go to Reiki to facilitate the pain and energize healing. Reiki has been a protected, viable pain management tool that might be a possibility for others. While choosing a practitioner make certain to check qualifications, get referrals and so forth pretty much as you would a physical therapist.

Stress Relief

Stress has different causes and can be investigated from different points of view.

From a physical point of view, stress causes blood to hurry to the extremities, and empowers the apprehensive, endocrine, and resistant frameworks. While there is a possibility that the fleeting impacts of stress may be extremely valuable, on the off chance that we experience a tiger for instance, the short and long haul impacts of stress in present day life are to a great extent simply adverse. A straightforward Google hunt will give us a not insignificant list of the diseases and disorders brought on by respective stress.

From a passionate point of view, stress happens on the grounds that we feel that we are at some level, incapable of handling a situation. Nature implied for stress to help us in life-threatening situations in the wilderness. We don't live in the woods any longer, and it is just when we intentionally or intuitively see a situation as a risk, that we feel stressed.

An understanding of our vitality frameworks will show us that stress is just conceivable when our vitality bodies are feeble. A few parts of cutting edge life, for example, traveling, television, PCs and the internet, computer games, garbage sustenance, and so forth prompt in increase noticeable all around component in our bodies. This implies every situation influences us profoundly, leaving us powerless to stress, and dejection and an absence of association with our friends and family.

At the point when people come to us for a transient arrangement, we help our customers by working on these levels. Reiki is scientifically turned out to be compelling in stress diminishment and management, in reducing the circulatory strain and rate of heartbeats and boosting the safe framework. We utilize hypnotherapy or vitality work to offset the feelings and the vitality bodies, strengthening a man's resistance to stressful situations.

For a long haul answer for stress, it is best to learn and hone Reiki on oneself. Reiki enhances physical health and passionate and mental agility, which enhance your proficiency at work, as well as increase the level of quiet one experience in day by day life.

Chapter 12: Mental And Emotional Healing

Mindfulness

Historically in the Reiki tradition, the use of mindfulness is absolutely necessary even beginning in the first degree of training, but it is emphasized even more so in the second degree, due to the intense nature of training in the advanced level. So what exactly is mindfulness? It is being conscious and aware during the present moment. That moment may last as long as a single breath, it may last for a full hour of meditation, or it may be something you strive for in every waking moment of your life. Because our lives are only made up of a collection of individual breaths, there is no better way to celebrate and appreciate your life more fully than by being conscious of each one of those. What has already happened is no longer your life. It is gone. I hope you appreciated it. What will happen is not your life. It is a creation of your imagination. Don't you want a life even better than you can possibly imagine? Then do not waste your time imagining so small. Exist in the here and now and you will experience it when it comes.

It is important to note that mindfulness is not an end goal to arrive at, but instead it a practice that leads you on a journey for however long you want to be on it. There is no failing at mindfulness; it is more about the effort to try. A crucial part of the practice is to come back to mindfulness after falling off track. Whether that means breathing mindfully, getting lost in thought, and then coming back to the breath, or if that means stopping yourself mid-word when you realize you are about to say something negative or that you might regret. These are all ways that you practice coming back to mindfulness, and in fact, is not a failure of mindfulness, but rather a part of its success.

Just like so many things we are discussing in this book, it is a skill that you must practice in order to improve upon. And just like Reiki, it is something that all of us already have and possess. There is only teaching about it in order to channel it. It is something that absolutely everyone can--and should! --do. It is accessible to everyone, and the benefits are enormous. Because it is a natural and instantly gratifying act, it takes little to no extra knowledge or effort to apply it. And because you are simply applying it to the life you already live, it does not necessarily take any time out of your schedule, planning, or special accommodations to include it. Nor does mindfulness require that you commit to some huge life change or acceptance that something in your life is wrong. Quite the contrary, in fact. A key tenet of mindfulness is that you accept and come to terms with exactly the truth of the moment, without any type of judgment at all. There are no comparisons as to what is right or wrong, good or bad, or choosing what needs improvements. There is simply deeply contentedness of acceptance.

Because the act of being present in the moment is a difficult challenge, especially at first, it will take some practice before you are able to be mindful for more than a fleeting moment at a time. That is quite all right. But you will notice, the more you practice, the easier it becomes and the longer those moments will last.

As a Reiki practitioner, mindfulness should become a way of life for you. Again, it is not necessary that you are perfect at it and never fall off track. In fact, if you were able to be totally mindful at all times, you may just be considered to be the second coming of Buddha. Short of that, that makes you a mere mortal like the rest of us, and perfection is not necessary. According to some, the simple act of being mindful, present, and aware of each moment is considered the absolute meaning of life. This means that each thought you have, each movement you make, each intention you set is done so with a consciousness and determination that imparts an almost spiritual-level of support behind it. It means that in every moment you are accepting of what is. You are not ruminating in the past. You are not worrying about the future. You are not wishing that things were different. You are not upset by things that you cannot change. You are not reactionary to outside stimuli. You are not swept away by your emotions.

All of that being said, you might have noticed that mindfulness sounds a lot like the amount of attention it takes to practice Reiki. That is exactly correct! Mindfulness and Reiki go hand-in-hand; not because they are the same thing, but because they utilize the same kind of "muscles." While it is amazingly beneficial, it is not necessary that you sit in meditation in order to perform Reiki. In fact, Reiki is a type of mindfulness, because you are focusing on the life source coursing through the Earth and your body. Applying the conscious thought is absolutely crucial to the art of healing by laying hands because while you are doing so, you cannot be focused on the results of your healing, how great you will feel after, or what you expect to happen as a result of it. These are all manifestations of your ego and are future-focused. That will distract from the mindfulness and make your Reiki less effective. There is no predicted outcome of any session, and to attempt to imagine the outcome is a form of pride in the face of the power of the unimaginable Universe's power.

Instead, when performing Reiki, either on yourself or another, it is of the utmost importance that you filter out all nonessential thoughts and expectations of what you are doing and what it might bring. The placing of your hands should happen with a clear mind, and that will assist in the blissful feeling of being one with the Universe. Allowing yourself to give over fully to the power of the original life source is the ultimate moment of mindfulness. It is the moment you will be most effective in channeling the Earth's energy, because you have fully removed yourself from the process. You are completely one with and in service to the life source.

Mental and Emotional Healing

One of the many benefits of using Reiki is to heal our mental health. This level of healing, however, requires being a second-degree student of the art. This area of healing is where we focus and are able to work with the conscious level of our thought process. Through this level we can recognize, alter, and improve upon our judgments, patterns, habits, and behaviors.

Because, as was discussed with performing Reiki on others, Reiki only applies as much healing as is necessary and the person is ready and willing to accept, this means that you cannot heal your mental health any more than you are ready to. So although it seems nice, you will not be able to become a second-degree Reiki student and instantly become enlightened. It will still be a gradual process that occurs with each new step of growth along the way.

There should be no concern over the efficacy or security of healing your own or anyone else's mental health, because as has been discussed in previous chapters, it cannot be manipulated for negative purposes. It does not resemble or act like any type of dark manipulation like hypnosis or spells. Again, it is merely the life source of the Universe correcting an imbalance, even in a mental capacity.

If you are interested in working with your mental wellbeing in general, you can do so by simply focusing your energy on a mental level. No need to have a specific goal in mind or challenge to overcome, but the mere act of channeling the life energy to improving your mental health will accomplish this. Through Reiki, you are activating the efforts and "muscles" of self-improvement, introspection, mindfulness, and self-care to encourage energy flow through these areas of your life. Much like physical exercise, creating a routine is crucial in building up your effectiveness and outcomes, even in Reiki. Through repeated mental focus of energy you will be more able to recognize patterns that you have, conscious or unconscious, reflect upon how those patterns are serving you, decide if that is something you want to change, and then brainstorm how and why you would change that.

You can also focus on specific problems in your mental capacity. This will require a clear understanding of exactly what you are trying to work through in order to best focus your energy there. The amazing thing about Reiki is, although you may notice an area you want to change, you do not have to know exactly how to change it or what the solution is. Because Reiki provides exactly what is needed in exactly the way it can be best accepted at that time, the Universe's knowledge will be all that you need. You can help channel more energy by using tools like the symbols mentioned in chapter one; you will need to become a second-degree Reiki practitioner to learn how to best activate these triggers. You can also combine these tools with the use of chanting, affirmations, or mantras. All of these can be done either silently inside your mind, or you can say them aloud. Either will work, but studies show that there is an extra element of healing vibrations that occur within yourself when you speak or chant aloud.

To become advanced in your Reiki practice, it actually requires a certain level of mental healing in this way. Because the channeling and focusing of the Universe's energy requires a certain level of enlightenment and connection with the Universe, this cannot be done with a closed mind. You must begin any Reiki practice with a certain level of self-awareness in order to harness the life force. One cannot possibly humble themselves enough to attempt to sue the original source energy of the world without this base level of mental aptitude and introspection necessary to heal one's own mind. The focus of our energy is reflected and manifested in our thoughts. Therefore, the more in control and focused your mind is, the more in control and focused your energy practice will be.

The Five Reiki Rules

There are generally five accepted rules to follow in order to get your mind the proper place for Reiki. These are general tenets that, much like mindfulness, are more about the journey of attempting them, rather than subscribing successfully to them at all times.

Today only, I will...

Not be moved to anger.

Not worry.

Humble myself.

Work honestly.

Use compassion in all that I do.

Today only, I will...

To begin with, all of the guidelines begin with the phrase, "Today only, I will..." in order to serve as a reminder of our mindfulness practice. The only time to focus on is the moment happening right now, and therefore, when it comes to our guiding principles, it only makes sense to focus on what is in our control, which is today only. To set a goal that is too grand or too large to accomplish will only serve to discourage you from attempting it. If a task seems too insurmountable to be completed, at the first sign of difficulty, you will have no reason to pick yourself, dust yourself off, and give it another try. Rather, these guidelines are built to do the opposite; they give you the very small, very manageable goal of not worrying about any other day. Not worrying about any streak of days going unbroken. Not worrying about cheat days or weekends. No, with these guidelines, you only have to focus on following them today. Yesterday is gone and tomorrow you can do whatever you want. Just worry about trying these things today.

Not Be Moved to Anger.

Anger is a reactionary emotion. Anger is not something one comes to after a lot of thought. It bubbles up inside of you uncontrollably, trying to take over our nervous system, our energy, our thoughts, and our reasoning. That is why the first tenant is to do our best to overcome this. We cannot experience life at our highest energy vibration if we are stuck in anger. This emotion usually arises from a disconnect between what you want to be happening and what is actually happening. Fortunately for all of us, we cannot control everything--or much of anything--so this is a responsibility we should take off our own plate. Think about it like this: to be angry about something that you cannot control is the ultimate example of fruitlessness. That is a lot of energy spent on nothing.

Not Worry.

Worry is an emotion-based in another time. Either you are worried about something in the past that has already happened that you cannot change, or you are worried about something in the future that has not happened and that you cannot change. Both of these instances mean you are not living in the present moment, which is the only time that matters, and is the only time that is applicable to Reiki healing.

Humble Myself.

To be grateful is to be humble. You cannot fully appreciate the gifts that are given to you if you fancy yourself so important that occurrences are rendered a nuisance. For that reason, you should try to humble yourself in order to utilize the massive force that is Reiki and be grateful for the energy flowing through you.

Work Honestly.

Integrity means doing the right thing all the time, even when you will not get noticed or recognition for doing so. It is that little voice inside of you telling you when you are veering off course, and it will not let you settle until you get right with it. To work honestly means that your integrity is in line with your conscious, telling you that you can sleep easy knowing you did your best. Truly, the only way to learn and become better is to be honest about where you are, where you want to go, and how you are progressing. The Universe does not have time for your ego-stroking illusions. It only knows and cares about the truth, so you should meet it on its level.

Use Compassion in All That I Do.

The ultimate requirement in Reiki is to have compassion. The life force energy that we are attempting to manipulate unites us with every other thing in the Universe. That means we truly are all one. The only way to use Reiki is positively, and the easiest way to feel the love and understanding you share with others is by showing them compassion. To honor and respect every other being's journey, struggles, triumphs, and energy is the most holy thing a human can do, and that is what Reiki asks of all of us.

Chapter 13: Symbols Of Reiki

As you learn more and more about Reiki, you will come across different symbols. You have likely seen similar ones in other methods, considering you may have seen Kanji in Japanese language. In Reiki healing, there are five traditional symbols.

Introduced as part of the Reiki system back in 1922, Dr. Mikao Usui envisioned the symbols at the end of his 21-day fast. It has also been said that their origins are much older since they have already been a part of the world while Dr. Usui was still studying what Reiki would become. Since then, the symbols have become essential tools in the world of Reiki healing.

The other symbols you may have seen in Reiki sessions that do not resemble what will be discussed below are classified as non-traditional. Therefore, they are not part of Usui Reiki system.

5 Traditional Reiki Symbols

When you aim to master Reiki, it is important to remember the five symbols that have been deemed traditional. These symbols represent the different aspects of Reiki, as well as how they can help you in your journey. They are seen as the keys that will open the doors to higher levels of awareness. As such, they are considered sacred and holy. In the olden times, they were not shared with the public. Nowadays, the symbols can be seen by everyone.

As you learn more about these symbols, take note that they do not hold any special powers. They function more as guiding tools for students and masters so that they can focus on the energy that they hold within. They are also part of the Reiki's energy presence.

Power

The "power" symbol, also known as cho ku rei, represents the increase and decrease of one's power. It is displayed as a coil and believed to be the regulator of the energy when it expands and contracts. Its intention is the light switch. Depending on where it is drawn, the power symbol can show the users its ability to enlighten or illuminate them on a spiritual level.

Harmony

The "harmony" symbol's intention is purification. Also known as the sei hi ki, it is used as a way towards mental and emotional healing. The harmony symbol is represented as a bird's wing dashing or the wave flowing across the ocean.

Distance

The "distance" symbol, which is known as hon sha ze sha, represents the intention for timelessness. It is displayed as a tower called a pagoda. Used as a way to send energy across distances, it symbolizes someone's ability to share their qi even when the ones they are sharing it with are not in the same physical plane.

Master

The "master" symbol, also known as dai ko myo, represents everything about Reiki. The symbol is displayed as a combination of multiple symbols and shows the users who have ascended their levels to finally become the masters. They share not only what they have learned but also heal when they are initiating attunements.

Completion

The "completion" symbol, also known as raku, represents the intention for closure. The symbol is displayed as a lightning bolt. As soon as the attunement is done, the users can now reach the completion of their ascending journey when they finally see this symbol.

How Symbols Are Used

Now that you have learned what the symbols are and what they mean, you have to know how they are used in Reiki.

Power Symbol

For the power symbol, it can serve as a catalyst for various purposes, such as purification and physical cleansing. It is also a useful tool for someone to increase their attention and focus. But most of all, it is commonly used when beginning a Reiki healing session to boost the practitioner's power. A good way to see how the power symbol works is when you are healing injuries. When you manage to cultivate the power symbol, it will be able to alleviate someone's pain and treat all light and major injuries.

The power symbol can also be used when one has the intention to get rid of negative energy. After all, it symbolizes purification, so you can expect to feel more positive energy when you make good use of the power symbol. This means that relationships, fortunes, and karma can all be purified with the help of the power you will get from the latter.

Harmony Symbol

For the harmony symbol, it can be used as a way for people to recover from traumas and past events that affect them.

Practitioners use it when treating addictions and depression and unblocking creative energies.

The harmony symbol can also help you achieve focus and retain information that you are trying to learn from various resources. For instance, if you want to remember all the things that you have read in a book or the Reiki moves without having to refer to too many resources, the harmony symbol is there to help you out.

As stated earlier, the harmony symbol works when you treat addictions. So, you can kick the old habits and cultivate better ones as this symbol helps you see yourself in a much better light.

Distance Symbol

Practitioners use the distance symbol to help people go through their personal issues. For example, when a person has an identity issue, it can guide them to be more comfortable with others even when they are not in the same room. It can also be used to bring energy from great distances. Though the receiver and the sender are not in the same physical plane, they can still feel each other through the spiritual plane.

Nevertheless, take note that the distance symbol must be used correctly in order for it to work. You won't get much out of it if you do not use it properly.

Master Symbol

For the master symbol, it is used to gain enlightenment. This comes in handy especially when Reiki masters are administering attunement to people who wish to become practitioners and ascend through its levels. Self-healers can also use the symbol to know how they can combine the powers of the other symbols.

The master symbol is considered as an important one among the five traditional Reiki symbols because aside from the benefits described above, it is helpful when you are doing Reiki meditation, strengthening your intrapersonal relationship, improving your immune system, and healing your physical body

Completion Symbol

Finally, the completion symbol is used to bring closure and rise with the awakened energy. It represents the ascension of a person from being a mere student to becoming a master. They feel a new kind of energy flow within themselves, which is something that they have never experienced in the previous levels.

You can utilize this symbol when you are about to end your Reiki session. You can draw or visualize the completion symbol and know that you have finally completed what needed to be done throughout the session.

The symbols are used by putting them on materials that can help the Reiki practitioners remember them while performing healing sessions. For example, someone can print them on posters while others can hang small tags as decorations. This is a way to let everyone know that the symbols are all around them so that they can achieve their goals and purpose with each session.

Still, do not think the Reiki symbols are used one at a time. You can actually use two or more at a time or even combine the symbols' powers to perform a variety of healing methods that others do not offer. An example of this is when you are sending Reiki for an upcoming event that's important in your life. By mixing up the beneficial symbols, you will be able to feel more focused and enlightened when the time is about to come.

Another example is when you try to heal someone from a distance. They might feel some kind of emotional turmoil or grief, to be specific. You can then combine the symbols' powers by holding an item that gives you a strong connection to the person. You will draw or visualize the symbols so that when you perform the healing process, you can send the Reiki energy and let the person know that you are doing it all with a strong and good intention.

In this day and age, you can also integrate the symbols in your life by putting them on your technological devices. This way, when something is amiss, you can check your gadget to see the symbols and remember that things will be alright. So, if your day is not going well or you just need a little breather, have a look at the symbols, remember why you are doing what you are doing, and tread on.

With the traditional Reiki symbols at your disposal, you can use them as you learn to master Reiki.

Chapter 14: Improving Your Ability To Channel Reiki Energy

As you delve deeper into the knowledge of Reiki, you will realize that there is always something to learn and so many levels of yourself that you need to explore and, sometimes, heal. Everyone has unlimited potential and with improved Reiki practice, you are able to tap into this potential. The key is to cherish and respect the practice of Reiki.

How to keep Reiki strong

Many people feel like they are unable to get the same results as they used to before when it comes to healing others or even themselves. It is possible that your Reiki becomes less powerful as you continue to practice it. In fact we all expect the opposite to happen. This issue of diminishing Reiki power is not related to any single type Reiki. Even the most senior practitioners of Reiki have experienced this from time to time. Some practitioners will tell you that there is no chance for your Reiki to lose strength and other will tell you that you are just as potent but your awareness of your Reiki power is the one that is diminishing.

However, if your clients are not responding the way you expect them to, you need to consider a possibility of a decrease in your Reiki flow. Attunement to Reiki is something that will last forever. What each practitioner needs to work on is maintaining the strength of his or her Reiki. This reduction of Reiki is not a frequent occurrence. But when you experience it, you need to understand why it is happening.

Usually, when one of your energy systems develops a stagnant area or some type of imbalance, your Reiki flow gets affected. Most often, this is the result of stressful situations that the person is coping with in life. When you ignore your own needs and focus entirely on healing other people, you will experience these changes.

Reiki consciousness works with the principle that all of us are essentially One. This is not some concept or philosophy but is actually something that you need to put into practice every single day. You need to maintain a good balance by helping others and then asking for help when you need it yourself. To make sure that your Reiki is flowing properly, you also need to make sure that you are receiving Reiki yourself. Self-treatment is one of the best ways to heal your energy channels, no doubt. However, from time to time, you need a hands on session with another practitioner, especially when you are dealing with stressful personal situations. If you have no other option, you can even receive distant treatments. When you receive a few treatments, you will see that your energy systems will just open up and your Reiki will get stronger.

You must always try to keep a balance in order to have a strong Reiki flow. If you feel low or unenergetic, make sure that you receive Reiki from someone else immediately. You may have friends who can help you. You can even join support groups for Reiki practitioners. You can also reach out to other practitioners to help them clear out their own energies.

Make sure you do not take your client's symptoms

Reiki is a form of healing. You are not really using your own energy but energy that you have derived from the universe or some higher power. Usually, the Reiki practitioners do not absorb any negative energies from the people they are healing. However, practice of Reiki in the west made it quite clear that this is quite possible. You can take on the symptoms of your clients. Many practitioners will tell you that they have had instances when they have absorbed the pain of the other person and experienced it themselves.

There are also several sessions when the practitioners feel like their energy has been completely drained out when the session is a little intense. This is a change in energies within the person himself. He or she could be doing this to himself or herself without realizing. You can actually open yourself to the energy of the client and the symptoms of his health issue. This normally happens when your personal interest in the healing session is not balanced. It is also possible when your own energy channels are misaligned.

Some of the most common cases when individuals experience the symptoms of the client are when their interest in curing the person is unhealthy. Most of them start out with the stress of generating specific results with each session. The practitioner begins to will for the client's symptoms to be passed on to him in order to heal or cure the condition. The practitioner does not mind giving up his own personal energy just to get the reputation of being a good healer.

When you are working on a relative or friend, you may seek a specific outcome more desperately because that person is important to you. In this case, it is likely that the practitioner will give up a large portion of his or her own personal energy. There are many instances when a practitioner will develop feelings of guilt for not being able to help a person the way they would like to. This is when they invite negative energies from the person they are healing into their own field of energy. This causes them to feel completely drained out.

All these energy exchanges happen at a very unconscious level. Your unconscious self is always looking for a specific result with each session. You may even be successful in producing positive results. However, the method is negative. When you have underlying goals or intentions, you create a pathway for all the negative energy to enter your space. You may not even be aware of creating this pathway. That is why many practitioners who take on the symptoms of the clients are unable to provide a clear explanation about why that is happening to them.

There are several ways to overcome this situation. To begin with, whenever you start any practice of Reiki, you need to make sure that you are completely aware of the fact that the healing should only be done by the Reiki energy. Set your own energies out of the way. This can be done by saying simple prayer before you start the treatment. Just recite the words, "May my energies be kept aside so that there may be an abundant flow of Reiki".

Next, you may utilize the power symbol of Usui and also use affirmations. Before you start any treatment, simply draw a symbol on your palm. Make one on each hand. To protect yourself further, you need to draw a large symbol in front of your body. Then, make smaller power symbols on every chakra of your body. Give yourself affirmations that drawing these symbols will not allow any negative energy to enter your body or field of energy. Tell yourself, " I choose to keep the negative energy of the client away." Repeat this statement multiple times.

You will be able to get immediate results with these methods. The best way to deal with any problem is to channelize all your energy towards parts of your body that is taking on the negative energy from your client. You can use Aura cleansing, healing attunement and regular Reiki for this.

You can use these three methods and additionally receive Reiki energy from another practitioner. That way, the process of healing and even the protection from negative energy is catalyzed. Lastly, focus on your own life and the different ways in which you deal with people and situations on a daily basis. Once you have been healed, you will notice that your

Reiki energy just gets stronger with each passing day.

Spirit release with Reiki

It is a common belief that there are several spirits that cause poor health and even other problems with your chakras. In the Bible, there are several references to Jesus healing people by casting spirits out. Even in the modern times, it is a known fact that there are several misguided spirits that can cause problems for people. There are several methods that allow you to channelize your Reiki energy to release these spirits. Each technique has a different effect on the release of spirits. You can use these techniques to release spirits or negative energies from people or even from specific locations. For this, there is no necessity for you to be able to interact with these spirits or even have any abilities of clairvoyance.

There are some circumstances when spirits are misguided after they have left their physical being. They will remain close to their home or even the people that they love. Such misguided spirits often fall prey to very low desires and will try to create problems for the people around them. The most common way a spirit affects an individual is by taking his or her energy away. In addition to this, they may cause poor health and even several other difficulties for the people that they are involved with.

There are several instances when a particular spirit gets attached to the aura of an individual. They can even get attached to a certain location causing several negative influences. A Reiki practitioner will be able to sense this sort of an attachment through the effect of his practice. He may not be able to clear certain issues for a client after several sessions. Then, the spirit release may be necessary for the client. This is an idea that most people will not accept. So, there is no need to discuss this with the client unless they have some inclination towards these subjects.

It is often assumed that advanced Reiki techniques will be able to help the individual. There is no situation where you will force a certain spirit to leave the individual or perform anything that may harm the person involved. Using Reiki is one of the safest forms of spirit release.

Spirit release is only possible when a practitioner has a very strong relationship with some higher being. This is possible with constant meditation techniques. Only an enlightened spirit has no ego and hence is able to release another spirit. They can work on spirits that are even highly powerful over the individual they are attached to.

You can develop this relationship by choosing a higher being that you want to build the relationship with. It could be a god that you believe in, a certain holy spirit etc. After that, you will meditate every day using a distant symbol. You will send out Reiki to this enlightened being.

As you say the prayers that allow you to strengthen the connection with this enlightened being, you will be able to experience their influence on your Reiki practice. You must mediate for at least 15 minutes every day for 2 weeks or a month in order to build this connection.

During the actual spirit release session, you will start out by saying out a prayer to the enlightened being of your choice. Ask the being to protect your client and also protect you.

First, you will perform Reiki on yourself. You need to draw the power symbol on your palms, in front of your body and also on every chakra. Assert that these symbols have been powered by the higher being that you are connected with.

The next step is to draw out the distant symbol. Say the name of these symbol three times and state your intention. The Reiki energy should be sent directly to the higher being. You will ask the higher spirit to heal and release the spirit that you are working with. These enlightened or higher powers are so powerful that they will be able to send the spirit out and release it completely. This ensures that the spirit will not be able to affect any being here on Earth.

Do not stop sending Reiki out until you actually feel the release of the spirit. There could be some residues of negative energies sometimes. This can leave a negative impact. So, make sure that you are constantly sending Reiki out even after the spirit has been released. Make sure you give gratitude to the higher spirit after the session is complete.

When spirits are attached to people, you need to understand that there are chances of the person attracting the spirit back into his or her life. This is why you need to make sure that the healing process is complete.

You can use healing attunement and aura cleansing to heal the person entirely. Using the distant symbol on the person can also help ensure that you are protecting the person with the enlightened spirit.

These methods of cleansing and healing will help you strengthen your Reiki tenfold. When you practice advanced techniques, especially, you will be able to feel the effect of Reiki on your life and the lives of people around you.

Chapter 15: Self Healing- Healing Yourself, Before Healing Others

Why You Need to Heal Yourself First

It is very important for you to heal yourself first. This is like, you teaching piano without knowing how to play it, or telling others to mediate, when you don't meditate yourself.

Healing yourself first allows you to experience Reiki first hand and to experience the long term positive healing affects that come with it. When you experience a self healing, you become energized, relaxed and experience a reduction in stress. You will see that your body appreciates receiving Reiki and the positive effects you will notice will be worthwhile.

The idea is that you will do self-Reiki every day. You might think it is a burden but it isn't. In fact I will help you more than you realize.

15, 30 or 45 Day Reiki Self-Healing

For this course you will be doing a 45 day Reiki self-healing, so you know firsthand, how Reiki can positively affect you. You will be advised to continue healing yourself, even after the 45 day requirement is over.

Reiki Self Healing Hand Positions

I find there are many different ways you can provide yourself Reiki. I have included the basic hand positions below for you, but if you feel guided to use different hand positions please do so as you are being guided to do that for a reason. I believe Reiki flows through our hands and they do not have to be touching together for you to receive Reiki. Therefore, if there is a hand position not shown here that you wish to use; please just follow your intuition and let the Reiki experience guide you:

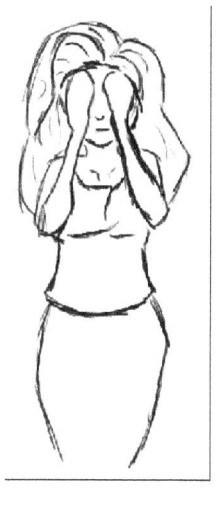

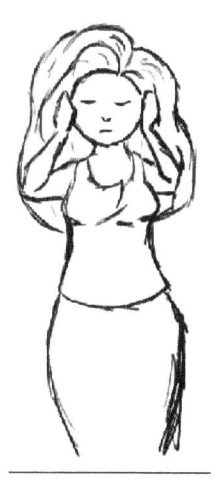

Self-Healing Continued:

Learning to let go

One of the most important things you can learn how to do is to let go. Letting go- whether it is of the past, a situation, someone hurting you, or just about anything- can clear your energy and make it more open for new energy. The healing that comes along with letting go is so peaceful and understanding. It makes you feel secure, loved and completed. It makes you feel less bothered by everyday life and it helps you heal on an emotional level.

By practicing Reiki self-healing daily, you may find that letting go becomes easier and that the "little things" don't bother you much anymore.

Healing on an Emotional Level

Everyone experiences emotional trauma throughout their life. Whether it is a childhood issue, parental issues or parental abandonment, maybe a loved one passed away or you experienced a rough relationship. There are many different life factors that can cause us emotional damage. By using Reiki self-healing you can use Reiki to heal your energy body and to heal your life in general. A lot of people who experience Reiki, whether during a session, attunement or self-healing- sometimes experience a release of emotion, whether through crying or some other expressive outlet. Reiki can heal your emotional self and release all of your past hurts, while replacing it with loving positive Reiki energy.

Being and Creating Your Best Whole Self

The idea behind this is that if you work to create the life you truly want and deserve it will make you happier overall and experience more of a positive life overall. What I mean by creating your best whole self, is that if you work on YOU, your health, your life, your career, your creative expression, your personal healing, your everything- then you will be creating a beautiful life, one that you have always wanted and it is also the life you deserve. Remember- you deserve the very best.

Nurturing Yourself on the Inside and Out

Nurturing yourself is highly important. It involves eating good foods, taking time for yourself, expressing yourself in creative ways, providing yourself Reiki and other healing techniques, taking time to read a book or article, taking an extra 5 minutes in shower just for you, taking time to play, taking time to go for a walk, and more. The more time you take, to nurture yourself on the inside and out- the better you will feel overall.

Let's face it, there is a high chance you are a very busy person, with stress all around you and even if you aren't totally busy or experiencing stress – you deserve to be nurtured.

Also, know that it is okay to accept from others. If someone wants to nurture you, or present you with a gift, or do something nice for you, or if they want to offer you help in any way- know that you deserve that and you should accept it with open arms.

Learning to Be You and Expressing Your True Self

With people all around you it is easy to be swayed to doing things you don't necessarily want to do. Sometimes you have to do work you dislike, or maybe your wardrobe isn't how you feel like you should be dressing. There are many factors to learning to be your true self and also to expressing yourself.

You, as an individual, have standards for yourself, you know what you like and love and you know what you want for all areas of life. Even if you don't think you know what they are, your inner self does and you can ask it at any time.

Learning to put yourself out there as the bright light you are can really enhance your overall energy and spirit. It will also likely boost your confidence which will help you improve your life as well overall.

Don't be afraid to express your true self- especially in the presence of others. They will love you. Expressing and being your true self- lets you shine like the awesome person you are. If you hide your light, how are you going to shine?

Figuring out what you want in life

This is something that was lightly touched up when we talked about intuition. Figuring out what you want in life will open up doors that you have never seen. You will experience happiness on many levels and be content in more ways than one. If you don't know what you want already, then you can ask your inner self to tell you. It knows everything from your life's purpose(s) to careers, jobs, etc. All you have to do is ask.

The reason I added this in is because sometimes we get stuck doing work and other tasks or jobs we don't actually enjoy. That sometimes makes us miserable, stressed out, and over worked. The joy we experience is diminished and our stress takes over our four bodies. But if we work to create the life we want and we actually figure that out- we can work in a job we love and genuinely enjoy- versus being miserable. Aim for happiness instead of settling. You can work doing what you are currently doing-even if it makes you unhappy, while researching and creating the new job- that way you will have the income you need while creating your new life and this goes for all areas of life – not just jobs, work and careers.

How to Incorporate Reiki into Your Life

There are many different ways you can incorporate Reiki into your life. For example, you can provide yourself Reiki while in the shower, eating breakfast, at work, during a nap. Your possibilities are endless. You can give Reiki to your beverages (except alcohol and other negative beverages/foods, etc.) and food items, you can let Reiki flow through you while doing Yoga, Qi Gong, Tai Chi, Walking, Running or other forms of movement and exercise. You can use Reiki while you are in traffic on your commute home, to help you get through a meeting, or family event and more. You can even use Reiki during social situations and the like as well. Reiki is a tool that you can use and incorporate into your daily life.

Using Reiki for Various Ailments or Issues (note: headaches, etc.)

You can use Reiki for anything. This is mentioned in chapter 2. Reiki is a great complementary treatment to any ailment- no matter if it is physical, emotional, metal or spiritual/energetic. Reiki is great for everything- no matter how small or big the issue is, or how long you have been affected by it. Reiki knows what you need and how much you need. Think of Reiki as your added source for healing; that can be a great compliment to any treatment you are currently using from your physician- for anything from headaches to cancer, letting go of the past or healing from an emotionally taxing relationship, depression, or just clearing energy from a long day at work. Reiki can assist you with just about anything.

Know that when you provide Reiki, that Reiki knows where to go, where you or the client needs it most, and it knows how much you/they need as well.

Usually, you will find that you intuitively know where to place your hands and everything associated with providing Reiki to a client. In some instances, for example, if the client has a headache and would like assistance with it, you can provide Reiki to them, but do not feed Reiki into the place that hurts, as feeding the energy into the pain, may not help but hurt more. Giving general Reiki to the client will help, in that the Reiki will effectively find its way to the headache, without direct contact.

How to Scan an Aura

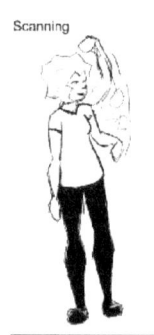

Scanning

Using your hands you can sense energy- whether it is yours, a pets, or someone else's. With your hands you can sense if there is a dip in the energy, which would be called a depletion of energy. This is an area you might feel intuitively pulled to place your hands during the Reiki treatment.

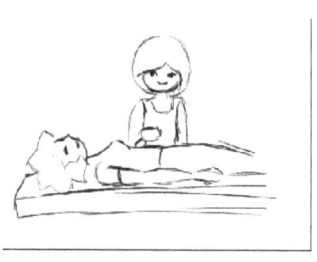

Place your hands, palms faced at the person or yourself. Use your palms to scan over your aura/energy or the energy of the other person. If you feel or sense something in a certain area- then you might feel like Reiki needs to be given at that area. You will sense depletions and other things, as: heat, tingling, cold, or no energy at all. Sometimes if the person has a large depletion, you may have to place your hands closer to their physical body to feel their energy. When scanning the body, your palms should be about 2-3 inches away from their physical body, sometimes up to 8 inches away or more depending on the person and how far their energy goes outward.

How to Clear an Aura

Clearing an aura can be done in many ways. These methods below can serve both you and others:

Visualize the person's aura in front of you / or visualize your own aura. Then visualize, with the opening of your eyes and the opening of both of your hands- the persons energy being taken over by a very large, bright white light. This can clear their aura or yours pretty efficiently.

Another way to clear an aura, would be to visualize a sea of Reiki energy going through their energy and taking any negative/stagnant things with it, and watch all that unwanted energy go out through their feet, while their whole body is encased in white/purple Reiki energy/light.

You can also ask your angels or guides to use a spiritual vacuum, inserted into their chakras, and gently vacuuming away any unwanted energy, then ask Archangel Raphael to replace the unwanted energy with Reiki or healing energy.

You can also do visualization such as a shower would wash away all the unwanted energy and the angels will take it and then ask them to replace the unwanted energy with Reiki or healing light energy.

How to Sweep an Aura

Sweeping an aura clears away unwanted energy as well but in one sweep. It is different than the

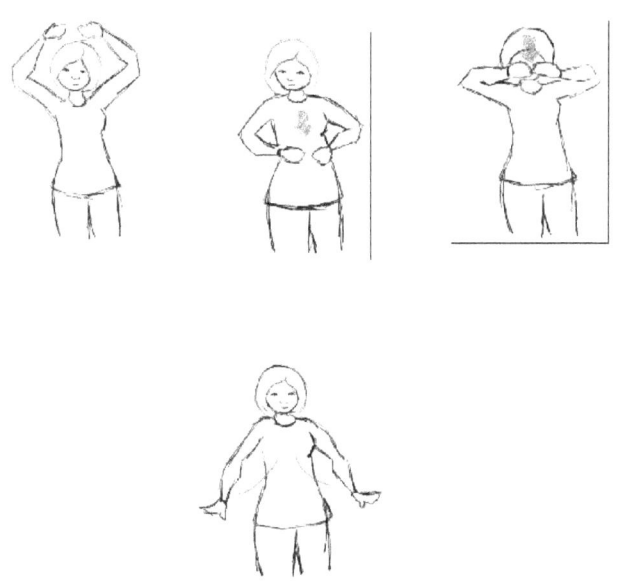

cleansing above because instead of the cleansing above, which is more similar to taking a shower if your dirty- sweeping energy is more similar to sweeping floors of dirt and getting rid of unwanted energy in that way. It is a great way to do a quick "once over" of the energy body during Reiki, or even just before you complete a session. Sweeping can also be done on yourself personally.

You can sweep yourself and others in the following ways:

Palms facing the person or your aura about 8 inches high over your head or the other persons head. Then make a sweeping motion from 8 inches above the head, all the way down their aura/body and sweep out just past the feet. All of this will be done a couple inches away from the physical body. The reason you sweep past the feet, is so the unwanted energy goes out and away from the person's energy and it won't get trapped near the feet.

You can also sweep starting anywhere- for example:

Shoulders down past the fingertips on both sides

Stomach down past the toes/feet

Pelvic area down past the toes/feet

Heart area, Throat or Third Eye, all the way down past the feet.

Crown/top of head down the sides of the neck, down the shoulders, arms and out past the fingertips

Lower back/back and down the back of the body, hamstrings, calves and out past the bottoms of the feet

Etc.

Keep in mind: you do not have to use both hands to sweep energy- all you need is one.

Chapter 16: From Patient To Practitioner

Interested in becoming an energy worker yourself? If you don't want to get a full professional license, and you only want to practice on yourself, family, or friends, all you need is first-degree training. Many people enjoy learning Reiki for self-care purposes, or to treat friends and family, even their pets! You do not need a background in healthcare to learn Reiki. In fact, even children can learn to be practitioners. By learning the techniques and principles of Reiki yourself, you can take time throughout your day to reduce stress, restore balance, and strengthen your well-being. You can use the techniques you learn to help you through moments of anxiety, or if you have a chronic illness, daily self-care Reiki can help you through times of pain.

There are three degrees of Reiki training, which are centered on attunement, education, and practice. They are as follows:

Reiki Level 1: First Degree

- This is the practitioner's initiation and is open to anyone
- Usually takes 8-12 hours
- Primarily experiential
- Overview of the history of Reiki, hand placements, and self or group practice
- Focuses on opening energy channels and connecting to the universal life force energy
- This level is more for self-Reiki to be practice on yourself
- Perfect level for the casual practitioner who does not want to become a Reiki Master and just wants to practice on themselves
- or family

Reiki Level 2: Second Degree

- Defined by practicing on others

- Students receive the Reiki symbols and level 2 attunement, which focuses on opening the heart chakra

- Students learn the ability to do distance Reiki, or the ability to send healing energies to people who are far away (students replace hand-to-body contact for mental connection with their patient)

Reiki Level 3: Third Degree and Master

- This is the level to learn how to teach Reiki

- At this level, practitioners have received the knowledge to attune their patients or students

- Some programs teach the Third Degree and Master separately, others teach it together as one course

- This is the level you need to practice professionally

Because all programs are different, it is important to do research to find the program that best suits your needs. While there is a set of standards that are taught across the board, courses of study can vary from teacher to teacher.

Conclusion

All in all, Group Reiki treatment is one of the options that can significantly enhance the overall experience of their clients. Some of the benefits relate to the clients where they get to experience a combination of positive healing energy from different people. The clients can also expand their social circles by meeting new people in the groups. Group treatment is also particularly effective when it comes to the treatment of stress and stress-related disorders. This is on account of its focus on both the curative and social aspects of the process. By engaging in group Reiki treatment, it is much easier for clients to develop a more positive attitude towards the process, thus improving the chances of success. From the perspective of the practitioner, group treatment can be a very cost-effective approach. This is because; group treatment reduces the amount of time that is spent on a single client hence increasing the number of clients that can be treated at any single instance.

www.ingramcontent.com/pod-product-compliance
Lightning Source LLC
Chambersburg PA
CBHW072010070526
44583CB00015B/1410